Plato and Potato Chips

by June Luvisi

Contents

Plato and Potato Chips

Prologue

I married John, my college sweet heart, and when he died last year, we had been married almost 59 years. He was ill for years. Having had two hip operations, one back operation and having been diagnosed with prostate cancer, worry had been a familiar figure at our house. When in school, I had taken a lot of psychology courses, and thought I knew something about worry and stress and how to handle them, but I found theory and reality are two different things.

Eventually the atmosphere turned very bleak, and I sometimes ran out of things to say to cheer up my husband who had to deal with daily pain. And I began to worry that both of us might sink into depression.

I started thinking about what I could do that might be a source of strength for me as well as a source of knowledge for our four children and thirteen grandchildren. I was becoming more and more familiar with blogs and considered writing one about my life. I was hoping that what stood out in my memory during the 80 years I've been on this planet might provide a kind of personalized peephole into the past. My granddaughter Sam assured me that I could write this new genre without difficulty and pointed me off in the right direction. Along the way, daughter Susan, son William, and grandson John have helped in too many ways to count. All of their enthusiasm and expertise spurred me on. This is what emerged:

Just Starting

Posted on June 25, 2010 by <u>June</u>

Hi, I'm here.

Discovering Mozart

Posted on June 25, 2010 by <u>June</u>

Mozart came late into my life. It was not until I was in my forties that the lyrical beauty and emotional pulse of his music began to talk to me on a personal level. As a young child I remember listening to a magical "Singing Lady" on the radio who would intertwine her glistening soprano voice with the excitement of a fairy tale. How I would run to hear her voice and travel with her to enchanted lands. My own mother had a beautiful voice and would sing as she worked around the house. She never had training, but she had a natural gift. However, I was born at the height of the depression, and she was focused on hanging on to our two flat rather than on developing her own talent.

Later on, Judy Garland would mesmerize me with her "Over the Rainbow" in the Wizard of Oz. Even later, Patrice Munzel, to whom I was introduced in a high school music class, would become an idol. Beverly Sills was another admired voice.

Now I listen in rapture to our own family sopranos. And somehow the exquisite fragility of soprano singing seems to me to find its most fertile ground in the music of the supreme master, Mozart. Even when it's not an opera, he makes the instruments sing. And my soul, too.

Just Sayin'

Posted on June 29, 2010 by <u>June</u>

For all you young people: If you think you know how fast time flies, be prepared. When you're in your "golden years", the passage of time can be like snapping your fingers!

Need for improved schools and Morning Joe

Posted on June 30, 2010 by <u>June</u>

God, how I love the morning! Especially this morning. Coffee, a perfectly ripe nectarine, a grilled Brie sandwich, oh, and some unbuttered green beans (to signify my good diet intentions for the day). I also hold good intentions to create a post on a daily basis, which I find is not that easy, given the interruptions of "ordinary life". Hey, I'm retired, right? So, a posting I will go. I saw a face on Morning Joe this A.M. that contributed to this exhilaration. It was the face of a man who radiated his passion for a dramatically successful charter school program in Harlem.

The program utilizes year round schooling, something I have long advocated. Everyone agrees we have to do something to make our schools more competitive with the rest of the world, and maybe this program should be studied in depth for patterns of success. The program is identified as the Harlem Children's Zone and it is led by Geoff Canada. We cannot look away from the deficiencies of our school systems, especially now when our children must compete in an increasingly global environment.

Truth and Beauty

Posted on July 1, 2010 by <u>June</u>

Oh, what is so rare as a day in July, today July 1, to be specific? About 70 degrees, sun washed air holding up a true blue sky, and yes this is a Chicago burb. I would compare this favorably with San Diego without question. Of course, Lake Michigan isn't the Pacific Ocean, but these days with the horrific daily reports on the Gulf Gusher, living near the sea doesn't have the same image it used to have. And we cannot forget the lush carpet of lawns, that holds our landscape in place. Yes sunny summer in Chicago can offer a beauty of its own. And as Keats said, "Beauty is truth, truth beauty". The older I become, the more I agree. Emily Dickinson expressed this so masterfully: "I died for beauty but was scarce adjusted in the tomb When one who died for truth was placed in an adjoining room, He questioned softly why I failed, for beauty, I replied, And I for truth, themself are one We brethren are, he said. And so as kinsmen met a night, we talked between the rooms Until the moss had reached our lips, and covered up our names.

My apologies to Emily for errors, but I typed the poem as I remembered it.

Socrates and me

Posted on July 4, 2010 by <u>June</u>

Socrates said," the unexamined life is not worth living", and I couldn't agree more. If a book I'm reading doesn't cast light on human nature, I generally set it aside. By reading about other people's lives, especially when these lives are convincingly conveyed on the page, I feel I understand a little more about my own life. Powerful writing helps me in my quest to understand life and put it in perspective. I think I have just assumed this would be true for most book lovers.

With this assumption, I casually asked a fellow book club member whether or not she too particularly enjoyed reading that enriched her philosophy of life. After uttering a flat "No", she looked at me as though I had come from another planet. This was a woman with whom I had been in a book club for ten years! Now I'm thinking that perhaps she found me more than a little naive. Perhaps she thought that someone as ancient as I would have stopped asking such questions long ago. After all, wise old Socrates said, "All I know is that I know nothing." Shouldn't I become more set in my ways? Perhaps. Just one problem: Can't do it. No way. To stop asking myself the big questions would be like trying to stop breathing. It's not in my DNA!

Plato, Mozart, and me

Posted on July 6, 2010 by June

What is called music today often, to me, sounds more like a roar of rebellion or a demo of notes rolled around in the latest vocal fashion. Of course, I know this immediately sets me up as an old fogey critic. But hey, it's not as though my definition of music is just the product of my "Donna Reed" generation. Plato said, "Music is a moral law. It gives soul to the universe, wings to the mind, flight to the imagination, and charm and gaiety to life and to everything." And if you dismiss this as Platonic romanticism, consider Nietzsche's assessment that "Without music life would be an error." Plato and Nietzsche would, I feel, agree that the most brilliant musician and composer who ever lived would be the divine Mozart. He performed as a child prodigy, and continued to play and compose until he died at the tragically young age of 35. And since he was on familiar terms with many of the high and mighty of his world, won many awards and generally displayed his phenomenal gifts to the power brokers of the day, you would think he would have had a relatively comfortable life.

Not so! Mozart had a lot in common with many of us today. He overspent in order to keep up appearances. He could not obtain a position that would cover the numerous expenses of a renowned artist. Though he worked feverishly, he could not get a job with a steady income and was dependent on temporary commissions. Struggling to pay off his many creditors, he could not support himself and the young family that he dearly loved.

To add to his misery he had to live with his cruel father's accusation that he had neglected his beloved mother when she was living with him in Paris and was responsible for her death. Sensitive and sincere behind his public mask, Mozart was pierced to the heart by such an accusation of irresponsibility.

Though I loved the beautiful movie Amadeus, I feel many have concluded that Mozart was a kind of clown as a result of seeing the film. They fail to consider the political scene in which he had to live and to understand that playing the buffoon sometimes deflected the social, paternal, and professional animosities with which he had to deal.

Mozart's true character is written in his music. It is there that we can feel the beating of his great heart. Plato would have loved Mozart. For Mozart's music does indeed " give soul to the universe, wings to the mind, flight to the imagination, and charm and gaiety to everything." Yes, Plato would have loved Mozart!

Gracious Japan

Posted on **August 14, 2010** by <u>June</u>

Sorry to say, it has been over a month since my last entry. I had a big problem with my back as a result of sitting in one position for too long. This time I resolve to be more faithful (and take more breaks)

Recently I activated my Twitter and have expanded my follower's list. I hope I haven't created any problems for myself, but I'm even using my real name. Couldn't resist expanding my world. One of my followers, a woman, writes from her home in Japan. As a result, some Tweets are in Japanese!

I have fond memories of my visit to Tokyo years ago. We stayed at the Okura and were treated like royalty. One day I wandered out on my own to explore the city and became so mesmerized that I lost my sense of direction. No problem. The first Japanese gentleman I asked walked with me until the hotel was within sight and courteously wished me a happy visit. Wherever I turned during my visit I found gracious hospitality.

Dog Days

Posted on August 15, 2010 by June

The middle of August in Chicago land. Dog days. Hot and humid. Yet having grown up in Chicago, I know such days are typical this time of the year. I remember living in what were called sun suits (think shorts with an attached bib) and downing icy, drippy Popsicles one after the other. No air-conditioning, of course.

We had a park district wading pool, into which I remember walking until the water was over my head, before I managed to have enough sense to walk out. You had to take a long bus ride before you got to a real swimming pool, and it wasn't acceptable in our middle class neighborhood to open up a fire hydrant and frolic in its spray.

It was hot, hot, hot. Yet we had one wonderful convenience: a back screen door. It was painted white, but it was so frequently used that fingerprints and weather had more than dulled its color. Weather beaten though it was, I loved that old door. Most importantly, it welcomed kids who might come to the door and call for me to to play. And when the weather was stifling, it allowed whatever breezes existed to enter our tiny kitchenette. We now live in what some would classify as an "uppity" suburb. The neighbors have expensive aluminum back doors that can stab you in the heel if your entrance is not speedy. Not for me! One of my favorite "amenities", and it was not easy to come by, my old fashioned, wooden, back screen door.

China and Grandma June

Posted on August 22, 2010 by June

Just a few minutes ago I viewed a discussion on cable that actually raised hope about our economic future! The basis for the optimism lay in one of the expert's comments that contrary to fears that China's progress will rapidly eclipse that of the U.S., China has reached the stage where they share many of the obstacles that confront us.

For example, the Chinese workers are becoming disenchanted with meager wages that barely cover living costs and are becoming more knowledgeable about environmental hazards. Added to this is the population decrease that creates fewer numbers in the work force. The interdependencies of Global Corporations were also cited. The program was Meet the Press, and one of the panelists was Niall Ferguson. The important point: China is changing so fast it is becoming much like us. Ironically, the more like us they become, the less likely it is that they will outpace us in the near future.

As for the far future? Time will tell. Well, at least there would appear to be a glimmer of hope here. I'll settle for that!

Wheels of Steel

Posted on August 23, 2010 by <u>June</u>

Roller skates. Wheels of steel that served as my magic carpet to bliss and adventure. As a little girl living in an apartment building, they were my passports to the surrounding world. Mother was busy with being owner, manager, decorator, and sometime janitor in our 19 apartment building.

The building was a ticket out of the poverty of the depression for my family. Mom was iron willed that the building would not fall into foreclosure. So that left me with quite a lot of time on my own. And even when friends could not come out to play, I had my roller skates. How I looked forward to tightening the shoe clamps (the adjustable metal clamps attached to the skates), buckling the well-worn leather straps and falling into a rhythm that propelled me along the cement sidewalks.

Ah yes, the cement sidewalk. Both my nemesis and friend. I'd look forward to the patches of smooth, even blocks where I could glide along with pleasure, and braced myself for the old cobbled ones that challenged my balance. Oh yes, roller-skating on cement could be blood sport! And even after all these years, my knees have remnants of the scars to prove it.

The Organic Egg and I

Posted on August 24, 2010 by June

Since as far back as I can remember, I've loved eggs. Although I buy and eat only organic eggs today, it almost seemed silly to seek them out when I first started doing so. After all an egg in its shell has a kind of natural beauty all its own. And cooked eggs bring back so many happy, delicious memories. As a little girl, on Sunday mornings, I remember my dad frying up eggs and bacon in that cast iron frying that was blackened and crusted with age. Just thinking about it brings to mind the wonderful, comforting aroma that permeated the home. When I visited Europe, I learned that eggs for breakfast are associated with Americans. Especially, eggs fried sunny side up. It seemed to me that the Germans and Austrians tended to think of them as symbols of our culturally youthful naivete. I suspected they believed we saw life as sunny side up and we wanted our eggs that way too. And now we are told that that lovely egg can be a missile of death!

Is this really true???? Perhaps the threat of eggs to our health has been exaggerated. Yet for some time I have been thinking we would have to pay for placing profit over the natural needs of animals. The latest news has it that even organic eggs may be suspect. I'm off to check this out, but part of me still wonders how a lovely egg could now be a fatal attraction. Now, where did they say to go on the net to check this out?

Wordsworth, poetry, and me

Posted on August 26, 2010 by June

I think it was in fifth grade or so when our class was introduced to Wordsworth. Though my mom and dad were intelligent and very loving, they were not what you would call "book lovers". Poems were just what others called poems, and pretty much remote from the substance of my life. That is, until I met up with Wordsworth's closing lines in his poem "I wandered lonely as a cloud" "...and then my heart with pleasure fills and dances with the daffodils."

Those words hit me, somewhere deep inside, somewhere between my young mind and my heart. That cold, dreary morning on the walk to school, I also "lonely as a cloud" had been lifted from my dismal surroundings by the graceful shape and dazzling yellow of some daffodils. The pleasure of the moment was exquisite. And it was amazing to me that I could experience emotions that had been felt by a famous poet, emotions that had been expressed so wonderfully.

From that time forward, poetry had new meaning for me. Poetry wasn't just lines of verse written in accordance with established rules, as it had seemed to me at the time. It wasn't until many years later that I learned of how Emily Dickinson said she knew when she was reading poetry. It went something like: "when I feel as though the top of my head has been cut off, I know it is poetry!" Although I will be 80 on my next birthday, if I am lucky enough to get there, I have never found a better definition. Thank you,

Emily, for rejecting all those high fallutin', scholarly formulas. I understand what you meant, and you were and are SO RIGHT!

Potato chips, the girl down the block and WWII

Posted on **August 29, 2010** by <u>June</u>

Some may think living in an apartment building that belonged to one's parents might be a pretty good way to grow up, and it was. That is, looking back over the years from an adult perspective. After all, it was the largest apartment building on the block. Of course, like most kids, I wanted more than anything else to blend into the pack. Being a landlord's daughter, and living in a small apartment in our building (though it was first floor front, as my mother pointed out), did not make for a life I would have sought out.

No, I wanted to be just like the girl down the block. SHE lived in a real house that was surrounded by well-tended lawn and gardens. SHE had a mother who stayed home all day and twirled her daughter's naturally curly, blond locks around her fingers after the girl emerged from a carefully drawn bath. SHE could pluck crisp red and white radishes from her garden and offer one to me. SHE had a large, welcoming front porch with a comfy swing. And I noticed with a pang of envy that she seemed to have a pack of friends.

I vividly remember sitting with her on her front steps while the two of us carefully licked the salt off Mrs. Japp's Potato Chips before swallowing them. We were convinced we had discovered a new method of eating them that brought their flavor on our tongues to a new level. Little did passersby realize that the two little girls in sun suits on the steps were gourmands in the making!

A touch of harsh reality colors the picture, however, when I remember that World War II was just around the corner. Suddenly Mrs. Japp's became Jay's because Japp sounded just like Jap, and who would want to buy potato chips associated with those fiends with buckteeth who were out to kill us? The government told us these people were so dangerous to us that they had to be hunted down and thrown into camps for our protection. Yes, fortunately, as years passed this demonization of the Japanese gradually faded from the public memory.

But what a lesson here for me. My visit to Japan years later would, of course, confirm my positive appreciation for the Japanese people and culture. Actually, there are many things we could learn from them, including their awareness and respect for elders. Sure good for nothings are found in all cultures and old age is not a guarantee of character. Yet the expressions of courtesy for old age bring something beautiful into our lives, something sometimes missing in our growingly callous society.

And do you know something? Occasionally, I still lick the salt off of my potato chips. There's food for thought there.

Keats and me and anonymous

Posted on August 31, 2010 by June

Thank you, anonymous, for nourishing me with your praise. To tell me that my blog conveys truth and beauty and helps to make life a little less hectic for my readers is the highest complement I could hope for. It wasn't until it was later in life that I really comprehended the significance of the poet John Keats' words: "Beauty is truth, truth beauty, –that is all ye know on earth, and all ye need to know." (Ode on a Grecian Urn)

How true! When we read the large body of superb poetry that Keats produced during the twenty-five years that he graced this planet, we have to step back in awe! And when we ponder the works of the great thinkers in the course of human development, we come back to the wisdom of his words. Some may find this truth and beauty in the Bible, some may find it elsewhere. Sometimes this truth and beauty can be found in the smile of the clerk at the checkout counter at the grocery store, or sometimes, in the supportive words of a loved one, if we are so fortunate.

Keats' personal letters also reveal the astounding mind and heart behind his works. To know what he knew at such a young age and to reveal himself in such profoundly beautiful writings, what a gift to the world! And thank you, anonymous, for your priceless gift to me. When I wonder about the value of writing a blog at 79, I can savor your high praise. I only hope to merit it!

Strawberries and my mom

Posted on September 1, 2010 by June

Oh, how my mother loved strawberries! Strawberry pies, strawberry ice cream, strawberry cream filled chocolates, strawberry tarts, strawberry everything! I remember how she would wait for the peddler coming down the alley shouting strawberries, or at least something that sounded like strawberries. His voice would be hoarse from the repeated shouting, but we all knew what he was calling. When the price was right, and only when the price was right, my mother would buy them in quart sized cartons and make her memorable strawberry pie.

She would roll out her tender pie dough, fill it with the sugar coated scarlet berries, and then carefully interlace the narrow strips she had set aside to top her work of art. When the pie emerged from the oven, the color of the berries had changed to a rosy pink, and the glistening berry syrup ran out of the small diamonds created by the latticework and gave off an enticing aroma. I can still smell it.

Yet most of all, when I think of strawberries, somehow I think of strawberry tarts. Actually, these were tarts from the bakery. Talk about gleaming red perfect berries (often topped by an inviting dollop of snowy whipped cream)! Talk about having the oozing berries nestled in crispy, delicious tart shells! The tarts, purchased at the nearby bakery on North Avenue, became a dessert mainstay at our home when strawberries were in season.

Besides looking and tasting so good, the tarts made me happy for another reason. After my mom purchased that first apartment building, she started to make more and more trips outside our home. We didn't have a car when we lived in the two flat, so the trips to the new property were pretty long ones made by streetcar. I missed her, of course, and when she came home with neatly tied white boxes of those treasures from the bakery, her return spelled double happiness. I can see the two of us savoring the moments.

As time has passed, I've tried many a bakery in search of strawberry tarts as good as those my mom brought home. Found some very good ones, too. But something is always missing. Never do they taste quite as delectable as those juicy red strawberry tarts my mother and I shared so many years ago.

Piano lessons

Posted on September 2, 2010 by June

When I was around three or four, my mother showed me a cardboard imprinted with black and white piano keys representing the octaves of a piano. The details of this teaching device are more than a little fuzzy, but the important thing about it, of course, was that it worked! It really taught me the names of the keys and made it possible for my mother to teach me the songs in "Thompson's Book for Beginners".

The really amazing thing about all this is that my mother, herself, had never had any piano lessons. And it wasn't until I was an adult that I appreciated her accomplishment. No one ever commented that this was kind of remarkable. My loving mom had gone to a store, purchased a model of the keys along with the Thompson's Book, and taught her little girl to play the beginning pieces after she herself had studied them. As I said, my memory of all this is pretty hazy, but I do remember that I loved my mom's lessons and the times we spent together at the piano. She made the whole experience fun. And she taught me "Long, Long Ago", which I can play from memory to this day!

Eventually, after moving into the apartment building, my mother arranged for me to take lessons from an "official" piano teacher and I progressed to a slightly more difficult piece known as "The March of the Wooden Soldiers." It appeared that my piano career was really taking off when my music teacher announced that she was giving a formal piano recital in a nearby auditorium. I did practice "March of the Wooden Soldiers", but looking back, I don't think I worked very hard at it. I hadn't an inkling of what it would be like to perform a piano piece from memory, especially in such an intimidating setting.

I dimly remember sitting at the piano, playing the beginning of "Wooden Soldiers", and for the first time in my life, having my mind go blank! Ouch! When I think of the embarrassment, I still can fee the heat in my cheeks! Having attended a zillion recitals over the years, I know this is not all that unusual. At the time, of course, it seemed like the end of the world. It wasn't the end of the world, but by mutual agreement it marked a long pause in my piano studies!

The breath of autumn

Posted on September 3, 2010 by June

The hot, muggy days that began September are vanished. The air is sun-washed. The blazing yellow of the mature black-eyed susans along the fence still remind of summer. Yet there's no denying…autumn is hovering.

Dickens and me

Posted on September 5, 2010 by June

Even before I started school, I loved reading, but it was in my second year of high school that literature loved me back. My teacher was a wise woman who taught us to appreciate Dickens by reading him aloud. Having an opportunity to hear my teacher bring "A Tale of Two Cities" to life in the classroom set off my romantic imagination. I loved hearing her oral interpretation.

However, when I learned we would all be taking a turn at reading aloud, anxiety set in. I was about fourteen, having skipped a grade and a half in grade school (no one gave much thought to social maturity in those days), and this kind of dramatic reading was unfamiliar territory. Unfamiliar and scary. Some of the other students had stumbled on the words and I was petrified that they would remain buried in my throat when I was called upon. It didn't take much to frighten me in those days and my hands were cold and sweaty as I waited my turn.

Yet the overwhelming and selfless love of the dissipated English barrister Sydney Carton for the lovely Lucie Manette had set my teenage heart afire. Imagine, Sydney was going to the guillotine so that his beloved could be with his rival, the man of her choice! And when it came time for me to read, to my amazement the words I read aloud actually sounded pretty good. Unbelievable as it seemed, my reading turned out to be fun. Dickens had so involved me in his characters that my concern for them shone through my words. For a while my shyness went out the window, and I felt exhilarated. Best of all, my teacher caught up with me after class and said those special words, words I will never forget: "June, I think you should be a writer!"

When I went to college and had to choose a major, however, I opted for a degree in sociology. I believed I could do more for humanity as a social worker and was convinced an English degree was frivolous. It wasn't until many years later that I followed my instincts and got a masters in English lit and returned to my love of language.

Going back to university in my forties was an adventure! Even when the professors left something to be desired, reading the great masters in maturity was like food for my soul. Later I worked as an adjunct instructor at Harper Community for six years and that was another mind opening experience. My life became so much more satisfying when it included literature. Here I am, sixty-five years after that eventful English class and that wonderful experience with Dickens. And I am writing.

Home birth

Posted on September 14, 2010 by June

I was born into what was then a relatively new section of Chicago in the northwest outskirts. It was made up of neat rows of brick two flats, one after the other on the parallel streets, with commercial development along North Avenue. I made my entrance into life in an upstairs bedroom on a very hot June day after a prolonged labor during which the doctor accused my mother of not pushing hard enough to deliver me more promptly.

As it was later revealed, I was wedged in the birth channel sideways, so when the doctor pulled me out thinking he had grasped a leg, it was really my right arm. I was at first not conscious and my right arm hung limply at my side. Fortunately, though I weighed only four pounds, to my mother and father's great relief, I started to cry.

Over the years they told me many times of how thrilled and happy they were to have their little girl. I was told they carried me around on a pillow, so afraid were they of injuring me. Poor Mom was furious with the doctor and accused him of incompetence; however, suing was not was as common as it is now, so they dutifully massaged my arm according to medical advice until it regained partial restoration and we all went on with life. Though my entrance to life was challenging, I had a treasure not available to all: loving parents.

Riverview and me

Posted on September 17, 2010 by June

Are you a Disneyland enthusiast? Think you know amusement parks? To really claim expertise, you have to have gone to Riverview in Chicago, Illinois. My mother and father actually met there, as did more than a few Chicago couples.

I used to nag my parents to take me to this wonderland of adventure. Because that is exactly what Riverview provided: TRUE ADVENTURE! None of this gentrified amusement park stuff such as we have today! Actually, Riverview had something for all ages, from toddlers to elders. Although it attracted families and had a wonderfully festive atmosphere, it had a somewhat sleazy aura as well. There was an element of danger, and I was cautioned not to wander off. It was torn down many years ago, but I remember it well.

There was a section of the park devoted to small children where the rides were much smaller and safer, an area that included a tiny Ferris wheel with enclosed seats and a miniature tilt-a whirl. As I recall, there was also a pint sized merry-go-round and a train that could accommodate both parents and children. It was here that I began my Riverview days.

However, my brother was eight years older than I, and could go on the "real rides". How exciting it was when my parents deemed me old enough to ride with him on a regular roller coaster! I can still remember the name, the Blue Streak. Of course, this was the tamest coaster in the park, but nevertheless I felt I was accepted into a new phase of maturity. The next level to follow was the Silver Streak; the rails were much steeper and the turns more exciting. I was definitely progressing!

Yet I still had to look up to my big brother. He routinely rode on the highest and scariest coaster in the park: THE BOBS! This was accomplishment in capital letters indeed, and his name being Robert, it was even named after him! It seemed I could never hope to reach such heights.

And then one day it happened. I looked up at the white posts of the Bob's platform that seemed to reach into the sky and heard the delighted screams of the daring passengers as they twisted and turned in the clear blue air. I told myself this was the day. Yes, I could muster up the courage to stand in line without embarrassing myself by running away at the last minute, or could I?

As I waited on the platform, it seemed like eons before the returning roller coaster racketed up to a stop and discharged its passengers. This was it! Too late to run! I found myself climbing into the Bobs seat and looked around to see if anyone else looked as terrified as I felt, but everyone was chattering and looked as happy as pie.

Suddenly, the steel pole that clamped us into our seat banged shut and slowly, slowly we clambered off. Rickety, racket up and up. I knew the first drop was the killer, and my heart was racing. I closed my eyes when we reached the top.

And then it was as if the earth had dropped away and we plunged into the air, down and down and then up and up and then down and down again. The sharp turns of the car threw us to the side with amazing force over and over again, punctuated by the thrilling drops for which the Bobs was known.

And...before I knew it we were clacking back to the rides platform. A safe return to Mother Earth! A little dizzy, I climbed out and looked around at the other passengers ... it was then it hit me. Wow! What a feeling! I had stared death in the face and survived! "Look out world", I thought, " Here I come!"

Emily and the world

Posted on September 25, 2010 by June

Emily Dickinson is one of the greatest poets who have ever lived. Truth and beauty abound in her verse. And had it not been for the Rev. Thomas Higginson, who imagined himself a superior, she would be better known. The audacity of this man boggles my mind.

Yes I am a Dickinson devotee! Ever since I learned that Emily wrote some of her poems on paper bags in her kitchen, I've felt a special kinship with this great artist of the poetic image. Her works reveal so much of what this world is all about in a way that could never be expressed in prose. I think of her poetry often as I go about my life.

When I consider how she was treated by Higginson, I wish I could have been there to tell her the man must have been either jealous or an idiot to have deemed that her poems were "not for publication". Can't you just hear the man's pompous tone when he described her work as "remarkable, though odd...too delicate-not strong enough to publish."

Nature speaks

Posted on September 30, 2010 by <u>June</u>

My somewhat rickety back screen door still beckons me to the mystery of nature. This morning I scanned the cloudless blue of the sky, checking unsuccessfully for a cloud, and was about to give up when I spied a pale, wisp of a moon, a remnant of the evening. So delicate, so fine, so almost gone. So almost like the memories of this past summer. The last day of September. The top of the next door neighbor's Autumn Blaze is touched with fire, so much so that what I thought might be a cardinal feather was really a fallen leaf. Orange- red against the emerald green carpet of our September lawn, the leaf drew me on. To speculate, to dream.

Two nights ago I beheld a far different world outside my door. We had just finished dinner, and remembering that I had clothes to be removed from the dryer, I walked into the laundry room that opens up from the screen door. Ah, a chance to breathe in the early evening! The scene remains etched in memory: Though night had almost fallen, there was enough eerie blue gray in the sky to outline the windblown branches of the giant, old willow tree that grows on the northern edge of our lot. The whistling wind swept the long, sinewy branches into menacing fingers that clawed and bounced in the air. It was a scene worthy of the cackling witches in Macbeth. I closed the door, happy to return to the warmth of the house.

Soup for the soul

Posted on October 5, 2010 by June

As a child, the aroma of freshly made soup permeated our home. "Parsley, celery, carrots and potatoes," my mother would say, "You have to have parsley, celery, carrots and potatoes".

When she thought me old enough, I was sent to the local A&P to not only purchase the vegetables, but also to pick out a large juicy soup bone with enough meat on it to provide all four of us with a substantial meal. Butchers must have had a large demand for soup bones in those days because, unlike today, they were readily available. I remember that the soup bone meat took on the flavor of the vegetable broth, and the result was a really tasty piece of beef.

Even when times got better, I looked forward to soup days. And when I was down with a sore throat or an attack of measles, there was that pot of restorative powers brewing away on the stove, sometimes steaming up the windows. Mom was a purist about her soup. Its taste was to be savored for its specialness, which was sometimes a delicate kiss of flavor. Dad had more liberal views. He liked his soup with a generous squirt of (dare we say it?) ketchup. If there were food police to call, I'm sure my mother would have called them.

As for me, I was half liberal and half conservative, depending on the broth of the day. Mom had other menu items for stretching what she called "the all mighty dollar", such as neck bones and sauerkraut, but for magical, restorative powers, hands down, it was her memorable soup with parsley, carrots, celery, potatoes and succulent soup bone that won the day. I can still smell the comforting, steamy aroma.

Miss Sandholm and me

Posted on October 11, 2010 by June

When we lived in that nineteen apartment building that was my mom's "foot in the door" to her real estate career, I spent a lot of time just hanging around while mom did whatever was necessary around the building to meet the mortgage payments. Dad was working a 40-hour week at Western Electric, and when mom fired the janitor, she provided the building's services single handily.

I remember she herself removed a lot of wallpaper (which she despised with passion) from the walls of those apartments. "Why, oh why, would people want wall paper anyway?" mom would ask."Why wall paper when painting is both easier and cheaper?"

Removing wallpaper required the use of a steamer, and it was shear drudgery! One day, while she finished her steaming, I was waiting for her on the back porch, and I peered through the screen door into the kitchenette of the adjacent apartment.

That was the first time I saw Miss Sandholm, a pleasant faced, nicely dressed woman, who was seated by the table. In a warm voice that matched her appearance, she invited me in, and knowing that my mom thought very highly of her, I accepted. As I glanced around, a simply, but tastefully furnished apartment greeted my eye. It seemed to me that I was in another world. Though only a young child, I sensed the thought that had gone into furnishing these rooms and it satisfied something inside me that

I didn't know was even there. Somehow I felt comfortable. Somehow I felt at home.

The social worker

Posted on October 11, 2010 by June

I could hear the respect in my mother's voice when she told me that our tenant Miss Sandholm was a social worker. Both she and her apartment had a quiet elegance. Proper, but very comfortable.

One morning when I was about seven my mom asked Miss Sandholm to care for me while she tended to some business. It was late morning when I walked into her apartment, so I was somewhat surprised when she asked me if I would like to have a soft-boiled egg. Now in our household we ate lots of eggs fried sunny side up, and, of course, we had hard-boiled eggs (What would Easter be without them?), but never in my life had I eaten a soft boiled egg. Don't know exactly why, it was just that way.

So when I accepted her offer of soft boiled, I really wasn't sure what she would be bringing me. As it turned out, she served the egg in a lovely ceramic white egg dish, which made the ideal backdrop for the perfectly cooked shimmying egg white and the bright sunshine-yellow yolk. So perfect, so pretty. In my little girl mind, I felt like a princess!

Unfortunately, Miss Sandholm worked long hours. She lived alone and was gone from her apartment most of the day. I saw her only briefly after that. She probably never realized the impression she had made, probably never knew that she had given me a glimpse of a life hitherto unknown to me. Of course, I now realize I barely knew the woman and most likely romanticized her and her life style. However, many years after that, as a sophomore at Northwestern, I had to pick a Major. I picked Sociology. And I think Miss Sandholm may have had something to do with that.

Peonies next door

Posted on October 12, 2010 by June

While we lived in the apartment building on Fulton Street, friends were not always available, and I frequently found myself with time on my hands. Fortunately, the narrow cement walkway at the side rear of the building permitted views of the neighbor's large garden area. There in the late spring we apartment dwellers could enjoy viewing the neighbors' gorgeous peony garden.

The entire yard was given over to varieties of this flower. The fat, round buds would burst open to reveal deep, rich maroons, velvety pinks, and cloud soft whites. Since our wooden back porches were so gray and utilitarian, the sight and aroma of the glorious peonies in bloom were most welcome. Of course, as a little girl, I wished the peony garden were ours, not realizing that in many ways, it really was: A free gift of scenery we could enjoy every spring without the work entailed!

The Sound of Music

Posted on October 15, 2010 by June

We had gone to see The Sound of Music with Florence Henderson the night before, and here we were in this steamy bathroom. I was humming some of the tunes from the show and trying to recapture some of the magic and thrill of the experience. The tickets had seemed fabulously expensive, but after much animated discussion, my husband and I decided to go for it.

This was the first, live, top quality professional musical that I had ever seen, and the performance blew me away. The song and dance. The wit and wisdom that flickered through the dialog. The marvelous, colorful costumes and the dramatic effects of the staging and lighting. All of it was unforgettable!

Five-year-old Susan was in the tub covered with suds, her curly blond hair piled high on her head. This day we were combining the bath with a shampoo and little foamy bubbles were everywhere. Thinking of the music from the night before, I started humming "Raindrops and Roses" and trying to remember the words. My singing voice was not the greatest, but the bathroom echo helped a lot, and soon I intoned "Raindrops and roses, and whiskers on kittens, bright copper kettles and warm woolen mittens..." And before I knew it little Susie in the bathtub was chiming in. I thought we sounded pretty darn good! What fun! Well, the long and short of it is, little Susie grew up to be a singer, dancer and an actress and won the lead in more than a few professional musicals.

Maybe her grandma's genes kicked in too, however, because my mom also had a naturally lovely voice. And today, as her grandma did years ago, Susan enjoys a real estate career.

All four of children were offered music lessons and encouraged to practice and play the piano. Two of them, Pat and Jack, wanted to expand their horizons in other directions. Since piano lessons require that parents invest a great deal of time, money and energy, I went along with their wishes. Pat focusing on getting a law degree and Jack focusing on sports and eventually running an award company. " Different strokes for different folks" was my credo. I never was a "tiger mom." I took Dr. Ben Spock's advice very seriously and sought to search out each child's innate talents and encouraged them to follow their dreams as best I could.

Son Bill plays the piano very well to this day and played it in various productions at Maine South High School. He was music director there and he even had his own band during his high school years. I think my mom's piano lessons, those lessons she could only give to me after teaching herself, filtered down like sunshine over the years. I don't think we're all meant to be musicians, but we can all appreciate music!

Streetcars

Posted on October 19, 2010 by June

Whatever happened to streetcars? I've always been fond of them, and I've never understood why they vanished from the streets of Chicago. As a young child they seemed to be a permanent fixture of life. Our jangly, bangly North Avenue streetcars were red and they could take you almost anywhere, if there was room for you, that is. Because at rush hours, a good sampling of humanity could be seen dangling from their rear platforms, hanging on for dear life.

Young men often climbed on at the last minute in spite of the conductor's shouted warning that the car was filled to capacity. And some not quite so young, too. Even women sometimes. I always thought the hangers-on had the most fun and envied their prowess. For streetcars provided a small public arena, a chance to show the world you were up to its challenges. Such an opportunity! And isn't this what most of us are looking for? A chance to be noticed, sometimes even if on-lookers might think us foolish or foolhardy?

As the streetcar made its way down the tracks, everyone who climbed aboard often had to grab onto a strap or, better yet, a metal pole to steady themselves against the sudden lurching that was a familiar part of the ride.

Once on board, you had better come up with the fare! The conductor stood at a substantial metal rail at the center of the rear entry ready to take your fare of a dime or quarter while balancing himself against the constant lurching. He could usually make change if necessary, but anything over a dollar bill was not viewed favorably. Around his waist he wore a shiny, silver moneychanger that chinged when it spewed forth its coins, and you could not pass his domain without payment. Or else! If someone tried to sneak through by melding with the crowd, woe onto him or her!

I've always been a people watcher and I found rubbing elbows with the public on streetcars fascinating. It stimulated my imagination, and to me it seemed as if the North Avenue streetcar at the end of the block could take me anywhere in the world. It could even take me to my own Chicago " ocean" (after a little walking). It could take me to our fascinating North Avenue Beach where I could see almost any kind of human being on this planet on the sandy shores of our beautiful and powerful Lake Michigan.

Corner drugstore

Posted on October 23, 2010 by June

When I was a little girl growing up in the 1930's, the drugstore on the corner was very special. It was directly across the street from the vacant lot where my older brother and his friends built a fort and played an expert game of marbles, no girls allowed! The store smelled of things like caramels and cough syrup, a distinctive aroma shared by most drugstores of the time. I loved that smell!

And what really made the drug store special was my big, loving escort, my dad. I still remember how he would take my small hand in his and proudly walk me down Mason Avenue, when he needed maybe some citrate of magnesia or some iodine or some Castor oil. I knew I would not leave without at least a piece of beckoning penny candy. The candy was displayed in cardboard boxes arranged on shelves at the end of the counter, and almost without fail my father would tell me to pick one out. Usually I would select a small caramel square that I would allow at first to melt on my tongue before chewing into its delightful, gummy center.

The trip was really special, however, when the walk to the drugstore was specifically for an ice cream cone! The amiable druggist himself would walk behind the counter and expertly scoop out delicious balls of ice cream from behind the marble topped soda counter that stretched over half the length of the store. He would then hand it to me, conveying to me a sense of adult importance. An enticing picture of the flavor of the month always hung from the ceiling and in the summer fluttered back and forth in the breeze of the fan. Sometimes I would opt for an exotic flavor such as black raspberry. But most times I settled for generous swirls of creamy, dreamy chocolate. (What else would you expect from a budding chocoholic?)

Today our drugstores in suburban Chicago are, of course, of the mammoth box variety, easy to get lost in and vastly different from the store at the corner. Bigger, yes, but for me definitely more than a little lacking in the unforgettable atmosphere of our corner drugstore of the 30's.

Radio days and "The Singing Lady"

Posted on November 1, 2010 by June

Before the magic of television, there was the magic of radio. And it wove its spell over us much like television does today, albeit in a somewhat kinder, gentler fashion. As a little girl of the 30's, the radio program, "The Singing Lady", provided me with a fascinating window to the world.

I remember my mother calling me to the radio when this fabulous dramatic actress and singer, whom I later learned was Irene Wicker, would be on. Her speaking voice was melodious and her lovely singing voice was equally mesmerizing. I now realize she gave me my first exposure to literate expression, and I loved to have her carry me off with tales of young girls shut up in towers, always to be saved by white knights who willingly put their lives on the line and battled the forces of evil that lurked outside.

Wicked witches and dangerous dragons abounded in her tales, and they were not softened by humor, as is the case so often today. As a girl of four or five, maybe even younger, I knew I was not being talked down to. This was quality programming. Ms. Wicker chose her sources well.

"Grimm's Fairy Tales" and Rudyard Kipling's "Jungle Book" provided fertile grounds, as I have come to know. And unbeknownst to me I was listening at times to adaptations of "the works of Oscar Wilde and

Charles Dickens" (Scoop, an e-newsletter). And I do remember how she would bring fairy tales to life so effectively that the characters seemed present in my living room. Somehow or other she would sing beautiful songs that related to her selected story of the day.

"The Singing Lady" was sponsored by the Kellogg Company, a huge name in cereal way back then just as it is today, one of the few brands that have remained a Titan over the many years. Yes, Kellogg's corn flakes, in particular, was a popular breakfast choice for many during the 1930's. I loved it with sugar and had to spoon it on my bowl of cereal because this was way before the creation of Frosted Flakes. However, I remember I was quite the Rice Crispies' girl, too, eagerly bending my ear to listen for that "snap, crackle, pop" that was so widely advertised.

Looking back, I realize that Irene Wicker was a true artist in her selections and interpretations of readings and in her beautiful and inspiring singing. She fired my young imagination and brought much joy into my living room on Mason Avenue. In our current, largely pop culture world, a program similar to Ms. Wicker's would enrich us. A program that would give our children a taste of lyrical music and literature. Not possible in this cynical 21st century, you say? I wonder. But be that as it may, this is a much belated thank you note from a little girl of the 30's to the " Singing Lady".

Edna May Oliver, Shirley Temple, and me.

Posted on November 15, 2010 by June

The other day when I sat down to the TV, I almost switched off an old movie from 1935 titled something like "Murder on a Honeymoon". I was just about to change the channel when I was taken by the intelligence and good humor that, even at a glance, was reflected in the face of the leading lady, Edna May Oliver. Well, how shall we say it, the woman mesmerized me. I stayed tuned in for the rest of the movie and had a great old time watching this woman interact with the other characters, always entertaining and clever, always lighting up the screen.

Now, I never would have known of Edna May had it not been for Ted Turner's Classic Movie Channel and I want to thank him for not only this trip back in time, but for many others. Just this morning I was enchanted again by Shirley Temple in "Heidi", marveling at the amazing warmth and keen understanding of the little girl with dimples who helped lift America's spirits during the gloomy days of the Great Depression. My mother was a fervent fan of Shirley.

In fact on my sixth birthday, she bought me a pink taffeta dress pleated around and round with rows of ruffles ala Shirley style. She had me photographed in this dress so I had plenty of time to stare at it and conclude that if maybe she saw some of Shirley in me, surely no one else did.

Mom spent a lot of time working on my mostly straight dark brown hair with a sizzling, hot curling iron, doing her best to replicate those gorgeous Shirley Temple sausage curls. And try hard as she did, the curls looked more like limp spirals than Shirley's bouncy golden sausages.

However, when I look back on this now, I'm smiling inside to remember her loving fingers as she attempted to give me the "on trend" look of the day. Mom was working long hours so she could hold on to our apartment building, our ticket out of the depression. So, thank you Ted Turner for bringing me an opportunity to meet up with Edna May though more than 70 years have passed since she starred in "Murder on a Honeymoon". Thank you for bringing Shirley Temple, the sparkling child star, to life again in 2010. And thank you for refreshing my memory of a mother's love.

Grandma June's Huckwheat Pancakes

Posted on November 20, 2010 by June

I'm not exaggerating when I say that it's been many years since we've had pancakes for breakfast. Though we're in our golden years, my husband and I try to eat today's definition of healthy, so buying pancakes from a box wasn't even in consideration. Yet as the November air has become a bit nippy in the morning, something has come over me that I could not resist. Yes, this morning I made pancakes from scratch!

If you don't like whole grains, this is not the recipe for you. However, my husband, who wasn't sure he wanted pancakes at all, gave my flapjacks a rave review. I stirred up the batter yesterday, so I only had to remove it from the refrigerator and it was ready to be spooned onto my preheated pan.

I used my Calphalon skillet and it served me well.

Grandma June's Huckwheat Pancakes

Mix together:
1 cup stone ground organic whole wheat flour
1 tbsp. baking powder
1/2 tsp. baking soda
2 tbsp. sugar
1/2 tsp. salt

Mix and then blend in:
2 tbsp. top quality olive or canola oil (I had extra virgin olive oil, so I used it)
1 cup organic unsweetened Silk
1 organic egg

Eyeball the pancakes carefully as they bubble and firm up.

Turn them.

Slip them on plates and serve with GRADE A 100% PURE DARK MAPLE SYRUP

We loved them, and hope you will too!

Mud Sculpture

Posted on November 26, 2010 by June

As I've said before, I was born in Chicago on the second floor of a two flat in a neighborhood of two flats on the far northwest outskirts of the city. The two story brick structures covered many blocks, but along North Avenue empty prairie lots still reminded us of what had preceded us there. We were provided a glimpse of Mother Nature in the raw, and even as a little girl I welcomed this, weedy tangles and all. I loved greenery. I remember being so very proud of the bridal wreath bush in the front yard when it was in bloom. So delicate, so graceful. So perfect for decorating myself.

And how could I forget those ever present golden lawn dwellers, the pesky to adults but beloved by children, dandelions? How many mornings did I spend crafting necklaces and bracelets and yellow tiaras made of them? It was easy to weave their sticky stems together and it was easy to pretend I was a princess when I had a tiara on my head!

However, even dandelions did not always abound. Our local two flats were all of an identical plan except for the color of the bricks or, more commonly, an enclosed back porch. The lots were identical in size as were the heights of the buildings. And sunlight rarely found its way into the areas between the buildings. My mother loved greenery too and tried to beautify this section with lilies of the valley. The lilies struggled with the intense shade and except for a few straggly plants and weeds, the shade won. My mother tried to water the lilies into life with the hose with only one positive result: an area filled with mud that had the consistency of cake batter.

This turned out to be a positive for me. What could be more fascinating to a little girl who loved to mold things than a malleable muck to fill toy cookie cutters and doll dishes? From little on I've loved art forms of all varieties, and back then this included shaping mud cakes and pies. I can still remember the delicious pleasure of spending many a morning or afternoon in my mud sculpture world, a world located conveniently between our two flat and the one next door.

The Cosmos and me

Posted on November 30, 2010 by June

I don't know about you, but I've always had a hard time picturing myself within the cosmic frame of things. And, just a few days ago, it got harder. I've heard that a new planet, a planet I call Oddball, has been discovered in the outskirts of space.

Planet Oddball does not rotate. This means one half the planet exists in various degrees of darkness and cold forever. The other half has constant light and must deal with the fiery heat from its star. No mornings, no evenings. Talk about a silent spring and summer! There would be no seasons at all. Life forms, as we know them, of course, could not exist... or could they? We are told that certain forms of life exist at the bottom of the ocean floor where there is no penetration of sunlight. Yet, on planet Oddball not only is there absence of sun, I suppose we can only guess at how cold it might be.

I'm not sure why, but the discovery of this unique planet makes it even harder for me to mentally place myself in the natural order of things. It is estimated there are 100 to 400 billion stars within the Milky Way Galaxy, and there are hundreds of billions of galaxies in the universe. Yet Planet Oddball seems to be the only non-rotating planet that has been detected. I'm not getting any younger and I guess certain things take on an importance they didn't have before.

Unfortunately, this non-rotating planet is so far away that I understand it may be eons before we get any really detailed information that will clarify the picture. Yet there is always hope when we have the Internet. ONE request! Please don't tell anyone I've named this planet Oddball. Star naming packages start at $25 and I'm not sure about the going rate for planets. I'm not looking for trouble.

Painting day

Posted on December 4, 2010 by June

Today I'm hoping to start painting this year's Xmas card. I'm fighting off some kind of bug, so I'll just have to see how things go...

Decided. I will be painting my three grandchildren from Arizona, who are now grown up, in a snow scene and carrying skis. It's a very happy threesome, and I like looking at them. Wish they lived closer.

It seems like yesterday when I babysat Jordan, the oldest. I can see him in his little portable bed when he was a tiny baby, both bed and baby balanced on the kitchen counter. A cherished memory. They have lived so far away, and I have only seen them a few times over the years. Maybe seeing themselves on my card this year will show them they are thought of with pride and affection.

I've already painted daughter Susan, John, Jay, Samantha, Emily, and myself in front of Susan's tree for a Christmas card. They grew up with us. Talented Jay took the photo that it was painted from and posed us. Grandson Wills was sketched in colored pencil on one year's card as baby Santa Claus. I hope I can paint more family before I leave this planet. Well, whether or not I can do this, dear family, please know that each of you is loved. You are part of me!

Motoring in southern France

Posted on December 8, 2010 by <u>June</u>

If you are ever driving through southern France, as we were about 20 years ago, don't miss staying at a very special hotel built on the foundation of a 13th century monastery that has been transformed into a beautiful hotel in Aix-en-Provence. I found it an unforgettable experience. Our handy travel guide-book had provided us with a map of Aix (pronounced X), and though weary from driving through the French country side, we felt confident that we knew exactly where we would find this "oasis of calm in the heart of old Aix."

The street was prominently shown on our map, and we could see ourselves quickly ensconced in our rooms, ready to explore this old city, a city where Paul Cezanne had done much of his painting. Cezanne is one of my favorites and I even painted one of his backgrounds in one of my own paintings. Finding the street on the map, however, and finding the hotel itself proved to be two different things. The street was circular, and we must have driven the long circle at least five times before we parked the car in desperation and asked for help somewhere near where the Hotel le Manoir was supposed to be.

A helpful Frenchman, proficient in English, quickly solved the mystery by pointing to a kind of alley that Aixians obviously considered part of the street. There, even visible from our car, was our elusive, quietly elegant hotel. "Ah, finally we could totally relax and enjoy our fabulous surroundings"! As we walked up the massive marble staircase from the receiving desk, I thought to myself of how cloistered nuns of the 12 and 13 hundreds, had trod these same stairs! Had he visited Aix, Chaucer could have walked up them!

Reading Chaucer in graduate school had been a mind bending event in my life. In his writings, I made what, for me, was a thrilling discovery: Though the language had changed over the many centuries, fourteenth century human beings were not all that different from us. Very recognizable personalities emerged from the pages once the Old English had been deciphered. I could see how sincere and not so sincere faith existed side by side. In Chaucer we find arrogance and vanity pitted along with some of the bluest humor I have ever encountered.

Human nature has not changed. The Canterbury Tales pulse with the familiar. Aix-en Provence brought back the excitement of really reading Chaucer! Later that day we strolled the Cours Mirabeau, the main street there, as I recall. I thought about being in the heralded territory of gastronomy and eagerly looked forward to partaking of a delicious dinner.

It was then that I noticed a seafood restaurant on a busy corner that appeared to be well attended. We generally ate only at cafes that were recommended in our travel guide, but this seemed to be a good chance to really mingle with the locals in this special city. And it was right in front of us, bustling with patrons. So we walked in and were quickly led to a table covered pragmatically in checkered oilcloth.

I selected a fish dish, recalling a memorable fried sardine dinner in Paris. And here we were in southern France, so often extolled by Julia Child herself! It was sure to be memorable. And memorable it was. It was about two hours later when I awoke from sleep with sharp cramps and a severe case of nausea. The onset was so severe that I didn't make it out of bed, much to my chagrin! There I was in a hotel built on the foundation of an old monastery, having climbed the marble stairs that Chaucer, had he visited Aix-en-Provence, might have climbed, and I had thrown up on this elegant old hotel's bed covers!

Chaucer, the father of English literature! Oh the embarrassment! In what seemed to be like the blink of an eye, an unruffled chambermaid was at our door, soothing my dismay with her consoling advice not to worry. "It's all in a day's work. Don't think a thing of it", she said. What soothing balm for my hot red cheeks! Several hours later, I was feeling much better, and we discovered an open-air market close to the hotel.

My appetite had returned (not a surprise in my case!), and we purchased an apple brioche that tasted like heaven. The rest of our visit was wonderful, in spite of this bump in the road. When it comes to selecting restaurants, however, a lesson was learned, albeit the hard way. Even in southern France, check out unfamiliar restaurants before entering! Those dining guides were written for good reason!

Christmas Card painting at the printers!

Posted on December 13, 2010 by June

There, it's off my kitchen table and at the printers. Little did I know about 10 years ago, when I started painting my Christmas Cards that it would be hard to stop. Know what it is all about? I've loved hearing such nice comments as "I keep a collection of your cards"." Never throw them away". "Are you going to paint one this year too?"

For a 79 yr. old Grandma, this is heady stuff. So when I thought about reusing an earlier painting, I couldn't shake off a feeling of giving in to the Grim Reaper's shadow on the wall. The next obstacle was that nagging feeling while painting that I might not be able to come up with a satisfying creation. Maybe it would be an object of derision, giving rise to such as: "Poor old lady just doesn't have it any more".

Well, people have the right to their opinions, but suffice it to say I think I succeeded in what I had set out to do. Anyway, it's done, finis! And as for that shadow on the wall?

Sunlight has taken care of that!

Oh, Xmas tree!

Posted on December 20, 2010 by June

Like me, our Xmas tree has undergone many changes over the years. As a little girl growing up in the depression, our tree was nothing to write home about. As I recall, it was an economy version of an artificial tree, unlike the beautiful ones available today.

It wasn't until we moved into the apartment building that my parents took that extravagant step of considering the purchase of a real live tree. "After all", my mother pointed out," A live tree is only good for one Xmas!" For someone who watched her pennies with a diligent eye, a live tree was an extravagance. And since mom made almost all the big decisions, that settled that. However, when the real estate investment started showing a nice profit, and my brother and I pleaded to have a "real one", she finally agreed, reminding us, of course, to shop carefully, lest the tree peddlers take advantage of us.

Without fail, it seems, the night of the purchase would be brutally cold. And without fail it would seem as if all the really well contoured specimens had been swallowed up early in the season. Also the balsams within our budget were in limited supply, and everyone knew that pines and other "exotic" varieties were quick to shed their needles or otherwise fail to fill the bill.

So in spite of the blustery cold and snow, we would continue on our search for the "holy grail", dauntless in our pursuit. We knew it was out there somewhere.

And we would find it! I can still feel the painfully penetrating wind that whipped us around as we made our mincing steps in the snow around the tree lot. But eventually our determination paid off, and there it would be. Our perfect tree.

Of course, we looked on our tree as family and excused any imperfections as assets that contributed to a unique beauty. Were there open spots devoid of branches? Ornaments and tinsel would easily hide that. And since I loved to lay perfect layers of glistening strips of silver one by one on the branches, even the barest spots shimmered in the glow of the lights. How I loved staring into its depths as I admired its magical glow.

Inevitably, however, the day came when we removed the lights and decorations from our perfect tree! The needles now littered the carpet and my mother had declared the dry tree a fire hazard. Looking over at its now vacant corner, I felt the living room itself seemed to mourn its loss. However, somehow life went on and the regular rhythms of life returned. I had some growing up to do. I would have to wait until next year, when once again we would seek out the perfect tree... I knew it was out there!

Full of Beans!

Posted on January 5, 2011 by June

So many people around my age treat organic foods with disdain. I don't get it. Yes, many of them are conservative types, but when it comes to what goes into what's left of this body, politics goes out the window. Take beans, for example. I used to avoid canned beans like the plague. I would dutifully soak and cook dried beans for hours in order to get a satisfying legume.

Now I easily open a can or two of organic beans, whenever the need calls. This is particularly handy for adding vegetable protein to green salads at the last minute along with high doses of fiber. Looking for a side dish for grass fed beef burgers or maybe bison hot dogs? Instant "baked" beans can be turned out by mixing with lightly browned organic bacon and onion along with a little organic catsup, mustard and maple syrup. And you know what? Once in a while the simple things are the best.

Bringing Up Baby

Posted on January 19, 2011 by June

With four children and thirteen grand-children, people might assume I could impart at least a few tips on parenting. I'm very proud of them all. But as soon as I try to provide words of wisdom for parents of today, I find it pretty hard to generalize. Each of my kids was and is so different, and I tried like the dickens to help each one develop his or her individual talents. Before you give me credit for my high aspirations and herculean efforts I must give a large portion of the credit to the oracle of parenting in the 1950's and 60's: Dr. Benjamin Spock.

Dr. Spock wrote a book that was packed with instructions and suggestions that came to be known as a bible of child rearing. I referred to this bible so many times over the years that even the second copy became rumpled and threadbare and sprinkled with dabs of baby food. There was one commandment that was threaded throughout the pages, and it was this: Thou shalt NEVER do anything that might undermine your child's self image! So simple, so profound, so all encompassing. And so, whenever I was in doubt about how to proceed, I asked myself whether or not my parenting was going to enhance my offspring's confidence. Simple, right? Well suffice it to say, it was far from simple.

Now, just yesterday, I heard an anchorwoman introducing an author of a new book of parental advice. The new book takes the parental role in the opposite direction from Spock. All activities should focus on getting straight A's and mastering musical or other cultural studies.

According to this author, striving for excellence should be the mantra covering all parental-child interaction. Case in point: your child has made you a simple birthday card that's been scribbled out with one or two crayons, say, one with a big red crooked heart with what could be little blue flowers. How to react? Whenever my own kids gifted me with their original works of art, often drawn on rumpled notebook paper, I received them with enthusiasm regardless of quality! Hey, if they had made them for me, they were quality! I warmly and gratefully thanked them. I put them on the refrigerator for all the world to see. It was what a mother did.

Now, going on 80, I hear my response could have been detrimental. Have to admit I know some people who actually pet their children in public. Ugh! Has a tiny sliver of doubt entered my mind regarding my own principles of child rearing? Had I at times mistakenly communicated my acceptance of mediocrity? Would they have become even better, more amazing than they are? Had I crippled their potential? Good grief, I sure hope not.

As to which school of child rearing is the best, you thoughtful, honest parents who really know your children, are in the best position to decide. Taking the time to try to really know your children is key. Most of the time you'll be right, but sometimes you'll be wrong. As my dad told me, when faced with life's tough problems, you simply do "the best you can". And may the force be with you!

My Dad's Hat

Posted on February 2, 2011 by June

So often when I'm enjoying a "golden oldie" on Turner Classic Movies I find myself looking at the hats that were worn and thinking about how much the hats reflected the social values of the times during which the movies were made. Men wearing fedoras always remind me of my father, who almost never left the house without reaching for his hat and automatically checking to see if it had the proper crease before positioning it on his head. In those days very few men (or women) left the house without a hat. A man's hat was a necessary symbol of his social significance. To this day, I cannot gaze at a fedora without thinking of my dad.

How different it is today! Most men go hatless unless a hat is needed because of the weather.

We have different symbols of social status today. Oh boy, do we! I remember how shocking it was to me the first few times I was checked out at the grocery by someone with a ring through a nose or a pin through a lip. It looked so very painful to me that I had to look away. Ow! I wondered why someone would want to greet the public with such horrendous displays in plain view. Today such mutilations are commonplace.

And then we have the tattoos. Yes, I know I'm 79; so younger people are not hunting me down to ask my opinion. But I cannot understand why anyone would want to have these designs etched into their beautiful natural skins, of whatever color. Yuck!

Musing about all this leads me to think there may be some similarities between my dad's hat and the piercings and tattoos. They're both meant to say, "This is me and I identify with certain ideas." In my dad's case, a hat identified an adult who outwardly wanted to conform, and the quality of the hat may have hinted at social class. However, society was such that everyone wore hats. Presidents and professors wore hats, but so did gangsters and men of pretty limited means. Conformity was expected.

In the case of today's body piercings and tattoos, the message seems to be: "No matter what you think, I want to retain my individuality!" Even though tattoos are popular among our jail population, and this would seem to be a deterrent, what proponents call body art remains popular with many. And this is true even though it's pretty generally known how extremely painful it is to have tattoos removed when they're no longer desired. Yet I wonder if tattoos might also be considered symbols of conformity too, symbols that identify the wearers as belonging to a "cool" subclass that remains critical of our larger society. They seem to say, "I don't care what you think, this is me! Nothing too scientific about this old lady's conclusions, of course. Just musings. Musings that started with remembering my father's hat.

Pops on the Corner

Posted on February 3, 2011 by <u>June</u>

Once upon a time, a long, long time ago, so far back that having a car was uncommon among a large percentage of the population, there were mom and pop stores strewn over the city landscape. On our Chicago block, we had our Pop's, which was located about six houses down from our apartment building. It was actually a small white frame home that had been converted into a candy-luncheon meat-cheese-you name it kind of store and, more than once it was a godsend in my family's life. To say it was a bit rundown would probably be an understatement. The paint was peeling on the outside and the wooden floor was leaning to one side on the inside. Yet I rarely found it empty. My grade school was located on the other side of the street, and when I would go there during the lunchtime break it was hard to get into the door.

With Spencer School directly across the street, Pop's did a landslide business in candy. In those days, grade schools like Spencer offered kindergarten to eighth grade education (an arrangement I feel is far preferable to the separate junior high systems that are typical today). There were lots and lots of students that stopped at Pop's to sweeten their day.

Colorful candy and treats galore were arranged in tantalizing display in a centrally located counter. To name a few: gigantic, garishly colored jaw breakers, ruby red and shiny black licorice twists, pastel candy buttons stuck on long narrow strips of white paper, black crows, red cinnamon coins, brightly wrapped bubble gum, peanut butter kisses, and my personal favorite, boxes of salty white-frosted pumpkin seeds.

Now as any kid knows, properly eating pumpkin seeds is an art in itself. First of all a decision must be made as to whether to lick off the salt or whether not to lick or to take a centrist position (lick off some, not lick off some). Then there is the matter of shell disposal. Those shells accumulate as quick as a blink! After these major decisions, however, comes the reward. A tiny thin pale green morsel with a flavor all its own.

In addition to treats, Pop's could be counted on for some food supplies such as popular sandwich ingredients. And actually it was at Pop's that I made my first important food purchase all by myself. Mom told me that we needed some sliced smoked pork loin and some sliced brick cheese. "Now, pork loin and ham are two different things, "she explained. "So you must make it clear that it is the pork loin and only the pork loin that you want." Her instructions about the cheese were equally specific. Mom loved creamy Wisconsin brick cheese. For some reason that she did not understand, store clerks thought Wisconsin brick and Muenster were interchangeable. While mom loved creamy brick cheese, she abhorred Muenster. "If he gives you a cheese that is colored orange around the edges, don't buy it. That's a sure sign that it's not Wisconsin brick." She then reached into the bosom of her dress, where she kept her cash, and counted out the money. And off I went, feeling very grown up, and more than a little intimidated by my new assignment.

There was quite a crowd around the counter when I entered the store, and Pops was trying to fill each customer's orders single handedly. It seemed he would never get around to taking my order. I think I said something like "sliced pork loin and brick cheese," and before I knew it I was being handed a neatly wrapped package and some change. With a sense of relief and accomplishment I scampered home.

Proudly I presented the package to my mom and stood there while she opened it. She unfolded the waxed paper and smiled at my purchase. There it was, so very neatly sliced that it made a pretty picture. Narrow strips of shiny white fat topped the pale pinkish pork loin. A very inviting picture. The slices of cheese were also attractively arranged. It could have been a food ad in the newspaper...but then my eyes went to the edges of the cheese and there they were. Though fine and delicate, there was no mistaking it: reddish orange coloring on the very edges of the cheese, annoucing it was Muenster.

Not a big deal to my mom. However, I guess it was a big disappointment to me. Here I am telling you about it, right? And I still wonder what my mom had against Muenster cheese!

Winter in Chicago

Posted on February 19, 2011 by June

It's a cold, clear February day. I just returned home from a spin to the bank. (Transfusion of funds needed!) The sky is a pale sapphire, and the sun is dancing along treetops and the newly displayed lawns. We had some heavy snows earlier in the month, and here and there are mounds of graying snow, stubbornly reminding us of what had come before. They bring to mind my looking out the windows of my home in awe at the silent white snowfalls, sometimes so thick they seemed an avalanche of feathers. I remember too the roaring cyclonic winds of that one true blizzard that had me wondering what we would do if the windows should break from the pounding they had to endure. I usually sleep through storms, but not that one! Now, viewing the cold brown, green and gray of the sun washed landscape around me, I feel good, really good.

It is a deja vu feeling that brings me back to earlier winters when we experienced similar snows and thaws. Except for trips to sunny climes, this is the canvas of my life. My mom used to say that we had the best weather in the country right here in Chicago. " Lake Michigan," she said, " tends to make the city cooler in the summer and warmer in the winter". Now that I've reached the "Golden Years" I agree. And call me crazy, but I think the absence of a change of seasons makes for a less than stimulating backdrop for life. California and Florida have their own special charms, but for me, I'll take Chicago!

Gray skies and stew

Posted on February 22, 2011 by <u>June</u>

Today the sky is as gray as a prison matron's uniform. Yesterday's cold rain has created a layer of treacherous ice that lies lurking beneath a fresh layer of new fallen snow. John, my husband of 58 years, has been told that he has lesions on his liver, and he has been having trouble eating. This morning he fell down in the hallway, and we had to call the fire department. They've been over a couple of times before, and they are a godsend in time of need. They ask the right questions and do their job efficiently, always with cheerful good humor and assurances that they are ready to help whenever needed. Here's a salute to these wonderful people!

Today John had one of the battery of tests recommended by the doctor. Daughter Susan took him over, and I stayed home and made bison stew. She doesn't need another person to steady and worry over while navigating the way to the hospital. Both John and I are wobbly as all get out. Actually cooking has become something of a challenge because I find it hard to stand up while I prepare the food. What I did with the stew was to sit down while the bison was browning and chop my vegetables. Fortunately my timing was on target today, and the meat was not over browned. My ceramic knife is a great boon to me when it comes to vegetable chopping because I don't need to exert as much pressure, thus enabling me to chop without painful hands the next morning. My stew veggies today were shallots, onions, celery; one small clove of garlic, mushrooms, carrots and potatoes. I flavored the broth with an organic bouillon paste and thickened it with whole-wheat flour. Later in the afternoon, John, Susan and I enjoyed a hearty, steamy repast after the hospital ordeal.

It was very comforting. And gray skies and stew, life goes on! Here's to you, kid!

More tests

Posted on February 28, 2011 by June
More tests. John is eating very little.

Filtered sunshine

Posted on March 1, 2011 by June

I saw the pictures. My husband has what look like fiery ulcers, an explanation of why he, who had a robust appetite, suddenly turned away from eating almost entirely? Time will tell, but it gives us some hope. If it is an ulcer, maybe it will be treatable. I feel so helpless. Must try to remember better days. Feel so helpless.

Stage fright, Act 1

Posted on March 1, 2011 by June

My big break in show biz came when my children were in elementary school. This was all because our suburban school had broken out of the mold of routine fundraisers by writing annual musicals. A group of parents wrote original scripts and song lyrics to suit each new PTA creation. I remember sitting in the darkened auditorium and gazing up at the performers on stage in awe, feeling I had discovered a magical world right in my own back yard. The parents had even constructed a home made marquee complete with flashing light bulbs that was on display for the whole world to see outside the school. Wow! This was almost too much excitement for this suburban housewife to bear!

Those people on stage seemed to come from a much more sophisticated world than I. The talented pianist thumped out engaging show tunes on the piano with zest and flair accompanied by an enthusiastic and expressive drummer. I was unbelievably shy, having bombed out when I was supposed to speak as salutatorian at my elementary school graduation. My mother and I had been late for the ceremony and I slipped and fell in the hallway, smearing my lovely dress with mud. I totally forgot my speech when I stood on stage, frozen in terror. For over a decade I was convinced I could never speak well in public. How I envied those parents who could shine out on that stage!

Well, a year went by rapidly. I was immersed in the duties of keeping a suburban household and raising four children. The next fall a note was sent home announcing the new PTA musical, inviting all parents to try out for roles in the new production. The memory of the excitement of that performance a year ago somehow outweighed those long engrained fears and I managed to talk myself into attending the audition. Parents ambled into the auditorium, looking very much at ease, but my hands were as cold as ice cubes. As you might imagine, it seemed an eternity before I was called on to read lines of dialogue. Actually holding the script in my hand gave me a sense of adventure that I find hard to put into words. We took our turns at reading accompanied by a lot of kidding exchanged between the regulars in the show. What fun!

Then came the scariest part of all: the singing audition. I was familiar with The Sound of Music and after looking over the songs from the show found that the song Edelweise with its limited range would be my audition choice. When I was asked to sing, I gave it my all and was amazed that the sounds were pleasing and in tune. The tender emotion of the song seemed to carry me along. Maybe I'd be lucky enough to get a minor part!!

To be continued.

Stage fright, Act 2

Posted on March 3, 2011 by June

My life in show biz via the PTA musicals lasted about four years, that is until our youngest child, Bill, graduated from 8th grade. So if my memory of one incident blends into another, please forgive. It was so many years ago. The feeling of heightened reality that I experienced still streams back to me over the years, however, and I am trying my best to relate it to you as I write.

The other parents in the show knew each other quite well, as I've mentioned. So I didn't have high hopes when I returned for the announcement of the castings. We parents dutifully sat in small groups sprinkled throughout the auditorium while the director passed out the lists of characters along side the names of those chosen for the parts.

Each show we did was a kind of takeoff of a musical, and this year the PTA writing committee had chosen "Guys and Dolls". I was unfamiliar with the show, so when I saw that I had been cast as Sarah, a kind of Salvation Army lady, I didn't realize what I would be called upon to enact. I didn't know that Sarah is one of the leading roles in "Guys and Dolls".

As it turned out I couldn't have been assigned a better introduction to PTA show biz. This role was in line with my own real life aspirations. I had originally hoped to become a social worker, and the part gave me a fun chance to live out my dream on stage, complete with navy blue bonnet and lengthy cape.

One of my character's important songs, I remember, was "Beat the Drum and Save a Friend"! I sang this while beating a drum with my Army, leading them around the auditorium and eventually up on stage. It was a bang up introduction to theater! Jean Simmons played Sarah, for Pete's sake, in the movie! Thrilled and scared at the same time this theater thing rocked my world!

Stage fright Act 3

Posted on March 4, 2011 by June

Wasn't it Shakespeare who said, "Life is a stage and we are the players"? Those experiences in the PTA shows do mirror a lot of truths about life. One truth underlined: In one way or another, we all like to feel important. I remember one afternoon at our neighborhood Jewel Food Store a week or so after the show. I was standing at the frozen foods cabinet when I noticed a woman standing beside me and staring at me. When I looked back at her, she said, "You were in the PTA show, weren't you?" When I nodded, she went on to say, "You were really good. In fact, you lit up that stage!" WOW! Right here in our friendly neighborhood Jewel. An honest to goodness fan! I'm sure I absolutely glowed when I thanked her!

Why was I so elated by her praise? I think I felt important on my own little stage of life. I didn't get too many compliments as I went about my every day duties as a suburban housewife, a mother of four. Her taking the time to let me know that she enjoyed my performance in spite of my nerves transformed my little world.

I try to remember how much her little comment meant to me when I encounter strangers who do something I admire in everyday life. I don't hold back my appreciation. On my Twitter page of today, I like to share my positive thoughts with my tweeps, just as they do with me. I'm finding there are a lot of people out there eager to make this a happier story that we actors are living out. Tragic and comic by turns, each of our performances counts as we strut across our stages. The play of our lives depends on us. As my mother used to say, " Life is what we make it!"

My husband's legs

Posted on March 29, 2011 by June

When we were going together at the University of Illinois I would sometimes have a chance to watch my future husband, John, practice for the U of I inter mural basketball team. He loved the sport and played really well, but at that time what I found most amazing were my husband's legs! Back then, in the 1950's, basketball uniforms included very short shorts, and I had a chance to study my boyfriend's hairy, muscular, and very attractive, manly legs.

The practice gym was located near the chemistry labs and I can still remember the smell of sulphur that permeated the narrow passageway leading up to the gym door. John was a chemistry major, and would eventually work in the labs of Universal Oil Products in Palatine, Illinois where he would be credited with numerous patents before he became an executive in the field; and when we were first married, many times he would plop down on the sofa after a long day at work, his uniform emitting that same sulphury smell that spelled lab.

So the memory of the chemical odor and the sexy image of my future husband in his short, short basketball shorts carries me back over time. There we are walking along the pavement in Champaign-Urbana, whipped by the blustery and bitter prairie winds, two young people in the throes of romantic love and blissfully happy in our togetherness.

John has taught me a lot about basketball, and we've watched many a Chicago Bull's game. The players pop up in person here and there on the North Shore. As a matter of fact, I almost backed into Omer Asik just yesterday at Whole Foods in Deerfield. (He was so tall that I had to crane my neck to see his young and sincere face. And, of course, I was too stunned to ask for an autograph!) I am a rabid Chicago Bulls fan in every respect. Love those Bulls! Have to wonder about something though. If push came to shove, could the Bull's legs match up in looks with my husband's legs? With these long basketball shorts of today, we'll never know for sure. But if a leg contest was possible and I could go back in time and enter that intramural basketball player that I married, I more than suspect my husband would win out. Yessiree!

John and his grill

Posted on March 31, 2011 by June

Hard to imagine, I know, now that one of our more common harbingers of spring is the aroma of meals prepared on our backyard grills, at least for us suburbanites: there was a time when an outdoor grill was considered an exciting new invention. Meals were prepared indoors on stoves and almost always by women. Betty Crocker in her red-checkered cookbook background reigned supreme, and I still have a well worn copy that I turn to, most often to check out the cooking time for a food. So early in the 1950's it was revolutionary to find the man of the house in charge of cooking all or part of the family meal. Suddenly, the black kettle of fire seemed to proliferate in every yard. Suddenly, it became essential to own and use this new emblem of "cool", the back yard grill.

And to my delight, my handsome, young husband took to it with relish! John became something like a priest as he ministered to his charcoal broiled meats and fish, cooked the properly primitive way above smoldering fires. The children, any guests and I would gather around the grill in admiration, often fighting back thick black smoke that stung and watered our eyes. It was all part of the ritual.

Ah, but what mouthwatering sirloins and T-bones emerged from his skilled hands. And no doubt about it: we were a successful American family. I had married wisely. My John had a natural knack for the barbeque.

Mountains

Posted on April 16, 2011 by June

Having been born and raised in Chicago, and not having traveled outside the state of Illinois until my marriage, for many years mountains were not accessible to me except in pictures. Yet I loved them without having seen them. When I drew or painted my landscapes as a young girl, I often included them in my backgrounds. They seemed to provide an extra dimension that was absent in my Midwestern prairie surroundings.

And so it was with great excitement that I joined in the planning of our trip to Colorado in the 1960's, a trip that included our growing family of four always curious, sometimes rambunctious children. All six of us would be viewing the Rockies at extreme elevations and crossing The Continental Divide! As we piled into our shiny, new station wagon, a tan Ford Country Squire complete with simulated wood panels, visions of lofty snow capped peaks danced through our heads.

Driving across Colorado on our way to Denver, however, the boring miles of flat farmland seemed to go on forever. Farms, crops and telephone poles and more of the same. "Are we there yet? "Where are the mountains, Daddy?" "It's so hot in the car, Mommy!" And I had to admit that it was as hot as the Sahara in that crowded station wagon!

We were really watching our pennies as our family expanded, and John had decided that air conditioning was an expensive luxury we could do without. When we purchased the wagon, for many people AC wasn't a necessity. Hard to conceive of today, but we were children of the Depression and it was a different time. However, as the hot, dusty air swooshed and whooshed through the open car windows, it was clear that air conditioning would have been most welcome on this trip! We had to leave the windows open. The temperature was in the 90's, and to ride in a closed car with the sun blazing away was unthinkable. It seemed as though we had found our own personal "dust bowl". And where, oh where, were those mountains anyway?

We checked our maps to be sure we had not gone astray. No one had told us there was so much flat land in Colorado! Finally, after we all had scanned the western horizon for what seemed an eternity, we spied some very hazy apparitions in the distance. Dared we hope that they might be low hills? It seemed like eons passed before we actually could be certain. Eventually, however, as we drove closer to them, we concluded that there was no question about it. We were indeed in the foothills of the Rockies! What a thrill for the six tired and rumpled occupants of that cool, "wood paneled" Ford Country Squire of the 60's! The real adventure had begun!

I remember finding ourselves in our first mountain canyon, of which there proved to be many, on our way to Trail Ridge Road and the Continental Divide. Numerous fishermen in high boots were intent on catching what I assumed to be mountain trout out of clear, crystalline streams that flowed over pebbles. Our road twisted and turned, revealing one beautiful gorge after another, scenes that might have been lifted from a travel magazine. The sun sparkled on the bubbling brooks and danced off the glistening canyon walls as we made our way ever upward, dutifully following the signs that promised we were on our way to the Great Divide, that high point that divides waters that flow into the Atlantic Ocean from those that flow into the Pacific.

Trail Ridge Road! Its very name suggested adventure! Beautiful scenery at every turn. It was if we were living a dream! However, in time we came to notice that the forest was gradually getting sparser and sparser as we made our way upward. Suddenly bright blue skies turned into gray skies, laden with heavy dark gray clouds. The temperature dropped dramatically, so much so that we reached for our sweaters and turned on the car heater. It began to drizzle as we wound our way ever upward. It seemed we were traveling on what looked more like a lunar landscape than anything earthly. Finally we saw a sign that proclaimed that we were indeed crossing The Divide and farther on we came upon an overlook and a shelter that provided information about the stark tundra landscape and some history about Milner Pass, a famous crossing point of the Rockies. WE DID IT! We had crossed the Continental Divide at an elevation of over 10,000 feet!

Though it was mid-day, it was almost as dark as night; we had to turn our car lights on as we proceeded to make our way back down from Milner

Pass. Our lights reflected on the shiny, blacktopped highway, and I found myself shivering in fear as we drove the curves of highway over what had become a black abyss. " Silly me," I thought to myself, "This is a popular and historical site. If it were dangerous, it wouldn't be open to the public". Still, I moved away from the window and did not look down.

The car seemed eerily quiet. I turned around to check the kids and saw that they had their eyes closed and were hunkered down away from the windows. Driving up to the Divide had been one thing, but driving down was quite another. With the highway pavement slick with a mixture of snow and sleet, and no car ahead to light the road, my heart was in my stomach. When I turned around again, I was in for a surprise.

It was then I noticed that there was a string of cars following us, and it suddenly dawned on me that my fearless husband, John, was leading a long string of headlights out of the darkness. I felt a swell of pride as I realized that our Country Squire was squiring a caravan of cars behind us. My husband, John, was our fearless leader descending the Great Divide, a leader undaunted by what driving challenges might lie ahead as we snaked around our mountain! Though I admit my eyes still avoided the windows, I felt much more comfortable. " After all," I said to myself as I gazed at my stalwart and handsome husband at the wheel, " We are all in good hands".

Lady Gaga and Mozart

Posted on July 17, 2011 by June

I've heard that Lady Gaga made more money than Oprah last year. Lady Gaga??? That cartoonish singer-dancer-performer who'll do anything to get our attention...words fail me...entertainer????

Well, there it is. Like it or not, the woman has become an icon of our age.

Before you dismiss this bit of information as frivolous, picture Mozart ambling along the streets of Europe and overhearing some one whistling one of his melodies from a newly launched opera. During his day, you see, for many people Mozart's music was the music of the day. His gorgeous, unforgettable melodies, his divinely inspired creations were the material of the contemporary music world.

His brilliant creations reflect his time on earth. As the world learned in the movie Amadeus, he had a deeply complex relationship with his stern sometimes-standoffish father.

Mozart, however, when he wasn't composing, loved to be out and about. Though the movie may have exaggerated Mozart's buffoonery, if you read the composer's letters and biographies, you soon learn he was a very fun loving and earthy man. A man who loved his wife and children, enjoyed the banter of his fellow artists, a good drink and a good time.

Mozart was very much a part of his society at every level. Having performed before the royal courts from a very young age, he had no illusions about the very real human nature of the nobility. He was as familiar with the high and mighty as he was with the common man, and his creations reflect his profound understanding of the human condition. Though he died at thirty-five, he was indeed more than an eighteenth century icon. His greatness extends to our present times.

Dare I, at 80, evaluate Lady Gaga as an icon and a mirror of our present society? Well, why not? At the risk of incurring the snickers of the young, I'm going to plunge my pc keys into her bizarre persona and try to shed some light on her mind bending success.

Yes, this old lady admits to being shocked to my Birkenstocks by the publicity antics of Lady Gaga. The Lady's dressing in raw meat fillets and wearing turquoise wigs of varying design has me doing a double take of disbelief. "Huh," I say to myself, "What is this world coming to?"

Why does such weird behavior appeal to so many fans? I guess I should know by now that the whippersnappers of today love to invert the perceptions and language of the past. A dress they like is said to be "crazy hot" or simply "insane".

"Cool" is one of those long lived superlatives that continues to be meaningful, but such carryovers from the past are pretty rare. Those whippersnappers want to make it clear that it's a new world we're living in.

The language of the past isn't capable of conveying the truth of the present.

One of the obstacles that I have to overcome is my strong tendency toward romanticism. I loved Doris Day and even liked to think I was a little like her. While I was on my honeymoon, I stopped in the hotel gift shop in search of something for a knickknack shelf. To my delight I spied a couple of loving ceramic bunnies with four itsy bitsy baby bunnies and was overcome with a need to have them.

I identified the shiny white bunny with pink ears with myself and I identified my husband with the affectionate brown bunny. Two of the teeny ceramic baby bunnies were white and two of them were brown. What a perfect treasure to display in our living room!

Over the years of raising four children, (two boys and two girls), those ceramic bunnies lost some of their ears and tails, but I still have the tiny, partially broken statues. They are sweet symbols of our romantic dreams. Throughout our marriage my husband and I would call each other brown bunny and white bunny respectively when we were feeling especially romantic, and we signed any cards we exchanged by our bunny names. If this is too saccharin for you, you may leave the room!

The music of our youth included many styles, but most had lyrics that you could understand just by listening to the song itself. Even our novelty pop songs like "Two Little Fishies in an Itty Bitty Pool" could be learned by listening to the singer. We knew what we were singing about. Today this is rarely true. Could this possibly be because life now seems so hard to figure out??

Lady Gaga's songs, when I look up the lyrics, seem to me to usually reflect an ironic look at life and love, a look, which, in turn, appears to express the prevailing attitude of the public. As such her music is art. Art is the artist's mirror held up to life, and life is partially molded by art. Yes, this lady fuddy duddy understands the success of Lady Gaga. Yet I worry about this old world that seems in many cases to laugh at romantic love.

Hot New Babymoons!

Posted on July 17, 2011 by June

No, I didn't forget to leave a space between baby and moons!

This has nothing to do with astrological spheres or astrological forecasts. What we're talking about here is a hot new trend of special vacations taken by savvy young couples who realize that hence forward their vacations will take on a whole new meaning and complexity. Drawing upon the familiar carefree conception of honeymoon, these young people are immediately calling their travel agent after learning they will be parents.

Yes, these smart, well informed prospective parents are planning babymoons to be enjoyed unencumbered by the responsibilities and restrictions that will shape future travel plans. These super prudent couples are so aware of what it will be like to travel with baby, they are scheduling babymoons patterned after honeymoons, sort of last chance to whoop it up trips.

Well, this sounds sensible on the surface, but maybe it sounds a little too sensible. We'll set aside the obvious need to spend money that may be needed for the incredible amount of baby equipment and other accouterments required by the new addition.

Having raised four babies without babymoons, I'm giving this moon thing more than a little thought. Would a babymoon have been like a second honeymoon for me? Actually I became pregnant on my honeymoon in the Ozarks so the honeymoon memories were still sufficiently vivid to quell intense longing for more travel.

However, the fly in the molasses for me was morning sickness, morning sickness that lasted all through the day and into evening and continued up until the last two months. I tried to remind myself that this was only beautiful Mother Nature's way of handling things, but I confess I became more and more critical of her system as time went slowly by.

The prospect of a babymoon would have held no charms for me. Oh yes, my veins were killing me, although I found some help in wearing the type of heavy elastic stockings worn by my husband's lovable grandma!

A glamorous fun filled babymoon didn't even enter my mode of reality! But these smarty-pants young brides of today don't seem to be afflicted by such yucky problems. They seem to be so much more in control of the whole pregnancy thing. In my day, we didn't even know the sex of our new babies until they emerged into the world.

There was so much about pregnancy that was simply never talked about in "good company". I remember the shocked look of the saleslady in our suburban store when I asked to see maternity clothes.

Obviously, I had stepped over the line of good taste by merely uttering the words! To consider displaying a pregnant abdomen on a magazine cover was unthinkable! Demi Moore would have been shown the door! Whew!

Feels good to have gotten that off my chest. Maybe it's the huge change in attitudes toward pregnancy that contributes to my reservations about babymoons. After mulling over the situation, the conclusion seems clear enough.

If a young couple can swing a babymoon in today's tough economic climate, I say indulge. If you think it will be truly pleasurable, I say moon it up! Raising a child in any age is a challenging job, as you will learn soon enough.

Addict?

Posted on September 5, 2011 by <u>June</u>

Okay, I am going to just steel myself and face this thing straight on. Am I or am I not addicted to checking out the latest on Facebook ridiculously early in the morning?

On a typical morning I watch "Morning Joe" on TV and enjoy breakfast in front of the screen. After finishing off that second cup of coffee, no matter how I fight it, I feel as though a magnet were pulling me to my computer.

Oh sure, I know I should dress and shower and otherwise be ready for the events of the day. I know I should "get it together "to create the "got it together" grandma person that I hope to project to the world at large. And now that I'm into my 80's, this "getting it together" is a major project! And major projects take time…. But…but… what if I miss an intriguing remark or photo streaming across my Facebook page? A little peek won't take but a minute…

Hey, hey…there we are…teenage granddaughter and I, just as we were yesterday at my son's home, she looking loving and lovely as she leans over and gives me a gentle hug. As for me, I have on my usual proud as punch Grandma look. Oh, and in the next paragraph there are my two youngest grand kids. Bright eyed and handsome, they look like poster boys for the Great American Family. What winning smiles! I couldn't have missed this! And then there are the other three children and the ten equally photogenic grand kids! And the nieces and nephews that I hadn't seen much of for years! Such fun to see their pictures from graduations and parties and new jobs. It's so interesting too to exchange comments with old friends and people who share common interests. As a friend commented to me the other day, the Internet Revolution will probably have even greater impact on us than the Industrial Revolution, and I love feeling that I'm a part of it.

So there you have it. This pull to the computer happens far too often not to detect there is a recognizable behavior pattern here. The truth emerges. The verdict is out. This Grandma is an addict of the Internet! I confess! It's an addiction I've grown to love!

Blondes Have More Fun!

Posted on September 23, 2011 by June

Let's see. You ask me about the highlights and lowlights in my life, the moments where I was most in touch with being me, just feeling good or bad about being in my own skin. Now that I look back, I see that many of these special moments were connected with…and are you ready for this?…my hair! Matter of fact, when I think about it, I can trace this hair thing back to my childhood.

As a little girl, I had a friend named Patti who lived down the street and who seemed to me to " have it all." Patti lived in a very welcoming home complete with a generously sized front porch and an old fashioned swing. I, on the other hand, lived in a three and a half room apartment down the street.

From my eight-year-old point of view, this girl had it made. She was a "golden girl". And what fun to sit with her on her swing and watch the world go by from her comfortable, swaying perch! What fun to sit on her steps and methodically lick the salt off potato chips before devouring them! Yes, Patti had everything: a comfy and well tended single family home, a mother who served attractively presented lunches and was always home and ready to fill her daughter's every need. And Patti had one thing that I coveted more than anything else, her beautiful, naturally curly blond hair.

I would sometimes be invited in after playtime to visit and watch pretty Patti being bathed and shampooed by her devoted mother. Picture a spacious, sunny bathroom with an immaculate black and white tile floor and, in the center of the room, an old fashioned shiny, white bathtub sitting on four curved, short legs.

Patti would be both bathed and shampooed in the tub, as I remember it, and her mother ministered to her as she knelt at the side of the tub. While Patti's hair was still wet, her mom would brush it out and then swirl a section of glorious strands around her finger. Presto, change-o, a perfect sausage shaped curl was born! In the blink of an eye, Patti's head was encircled with shiny blonde Shirley Temple curls, beautiful beyond belief!

This was the passion of the time, of course. Everything for young girls, from dresses to hair bows and paper dolls, was modeled on Shirley Temple; Shirley Temple curls especially were the epitome of cool. Mom did the best she could with a hot curling iron applied to my limp brown hair, but no matter how hard she worked my stringy spirals definitely weren't in the same league.

And when it came to dolls, they had to be blonde, of course. Or so I wished. You see, my mom had purchased a nineteen apartment building in the grip of the Great Depression. Money was tight.

I remember one Christmas when mom had taken me down to the Loop to visit the Fair Store's Toyland. We took the escalator up and up to the glistening floor of magical delight, and it was there I spied a beautifully dressed gorgeous blonde doll that I yearned to have for my own. I thought mom agreed with my selection, but when it was delivered and I opened the box sometime later, I found a tall brunette doll in its place. Mom pointed out how pretty the doll was and how much bigger it was than my first choice and how much CHEAPER!

Well… I can still remember how stunned and disappointed I felt. Some tears were shed. Money problems were not something I could get my little girl's mind around. Mom always made me feel I was cherished, so how could this be? As I see it now, mom probably thought a tall, pretty brunette doll would be welcomed into my doll family with enthusiasm. (And bigger, better, and cheaper had such a nice ring!) Well, the doll did move in with my other dolls, but she played a minor role in doll activities. I just couldn't shake this hair thing.

Thinking of hair brings me back to that era of more than a few years ago when wigs for women were almost de rigour. Somehow it seemed that overnight, every woman of fashion could not leave the house without a chic, well-aerated hairpiece. "Feather light", beautifully styled wigs were advertised everywhere.

This was a great opportunity for this stay-at-home mother of four to experiment with a new color. Have to admit I was too intimidated to suddenly go blond by wig. (Oh my gosh, what would the neighbors think?) So I took the middle road of compromise: I purchased a light brown wig that was silver frosted. Even going this far had impact.

Suddenly I found I was being treated differently by the outside world, or so I thought. I felt more than a little daring. In today's jargon, I felt "cool." However, it wasn't too long before wig wearing lost its status. I guess women came to recognize those "feather light" wigs were really not all that comfortable after all. Ah, but I was no longer the same person! I had dared to cross over from brunette to frosted territory! The door had been opened a crack.

And so it came to be that when I was on a vacation in Southern California, and had a much needed hair appointment, I was open to options. But when the sophisticated California colorist told me she thought I would find blonde hair brought out the color of my eyes, I could hardly trust my ears.

Imagine me: a California blonde! I took every opportunity I could to glimpse the new me in mirrors! The regular rhythms of family life still continued, of course, when I returned to the Midwest. But from that day on, though my roots of silver might belie it, I have lived my life as a blonde. And I have to agree: over the years, being blonde has often been fun.

Yet underneath it all, and dopey as it sounds, I have occasional qualms about passing myself as something I'm not. So you can imagine my reaction when old lady me was sitting in the waiting room of my favorite beauty salon the other day and another salon patron asked me if I was Swedish.

The golden threads among the silver of my hair must have caught her attention. She was just making small talk, most likely, but little did she realize how much her words were music to my ears. "Swedish? Hey, maybe I've pulled it off, after all," I thought…" What a nifty moment!"

And I've treasured nifty moments more and more as old age has intruded into my lifestyle…in my case arthritis has convinced me of the truth of Bette Davis's observation that "old age ain't for sissies." "Imagine that," I said to myself," this woman thinks I am a natural Swedish blonde!" So here I am, savoring that moment and testifying to that old adage about the advantages of living life as a golden girl… Yes, this blonde really has had more fun! Especially at eighty!

Chicago's Wondrous Weather!

Posted on January 4, 2012 by June

As I look out the dining room window at the bright sunlight flooding the back yard, I remember my mom telling me how lucky we were to enjoy living in Chicago. "Lake Michigan keeps us cooler in the summer and warmer in the winter," she would say. Mom loved Chicago with a passion, so I would take her words with a grain of salt. I knew she was prejudiced.

You know how it's said about New York that if you can make it there, you can make it anywhere? Mom said that she chose to go with more favorable odds. She believed Chicago offered maximum opportunity for success, and this colored her thinking about other issues at times. Over the years I've heard more than a few discouraging words from others about Chicago's weather, especially the winter. I had come to dismiss my mother's praise of Chicago's climate as excessive. That is until this winter. Here we are January 4, and it is already around 37 degrees, beautiful blue sky and sunlight flooding the landscape. The weather this morning is invigorating. It speaks to me and invites me to write this post. It's the kind of weather that suggests activity and thought... I feel really alive! And as I look outside at the trees and shrubbery, I see mostly green, and there is not a breath of wind to be seen.

Down in Florida the snowbirds are fighting off freezing temperatures. I can empathize: I remember being bundled up and shivering by the side of the hotel pool one winter in Florida and being stunned by the powerful winds and the frigid surroundings. I even wore earmuffs and mittens by that pool! Nothing worse than being ill prepared for wintry blasts. In Chicago we prepare. And a sunny 38 degrees feels good in January. The weatherman promises even warmer days in the near future... Erasing memories of snowbound driveways comes easy today. Come to think of it, even with snowbound driveways, I relish the familiar change of seasons. And this day there aren't any reservations whatsoever! This gorgeous January day, I'll take Chicago!

Grandma, a Geek!

Posted on January 27, 2012 by June

If you asked me this outright, I would assure you my answer would be a loud "NO!" I've always been a right brain person, always found myself drawn to art and the language arts. My grandson Jack, on the other hand, is a good example of someone who excels at technology and loves to familiarize himself with the rapidly changing world of technology.

His 21st birthday is fast approaching, and when asked what kind of new PC he might like for his birthday, he answered by producing a long series of symbols." What I would like, Grandma is to have these computer parts." In other words, what my grandson wants, instead of a shiny new computer all set and ready to go, is a box of unassembled parts with which he can build his own customized computer.

Now that's what I call an impressive Geek identity! It is, in fact, a little hard for me to believe. I have a love-hate relationship with my amazing Macbook Pro. At times I'd swear there is a little person in there who anticipates my needs even before I myself know what they are. At such times I am a user in awe! And then, of course, there are the other times. Such as when I wish to switch material from one blogging set-up to another.

Just the other day, I wanted to add a recent post from another format to my blog on Microsoft Word. I knew that one of those many little symbols bordering the page could perform the transfer, no problem, and yet nothing I tried worked. NOTHING! Fortunately, however, one of my offspring came over and saved the day. My face was a bit red and I have to admit, my need to ask for help took a poke at my ego. Well, this type of thing happens often enough so that the question can definitely be put to rest.

Grandma enjoys posting on her blog and sharing her opinions with the world, but no need to be concerned about her getting an inflated view of herself. The little twists and turns of her challenging tech world will not allow for that.

The unvarnished truth is that Grandma is not now, and never will be a Geek. (Drat!)

Chopin's Golden Years

Posted on February 1, 2012 by June

Some say Chopin was the most influential of composers of piano music. Like Mozart, however, Chopin died at an early age; he only lived to be 39. Hence you may be wondering how and why I could be writing about Chopin's golden years. Let me explain.

Recently I was treated to hearing one of his waltzes played by a wonderfully talented pianist who is in what we call our golden years. (Yes, I too am in this "golden" category.) She played the piece so beautifully that if he had heard it, I'm sure the great master would have been pleased. We were the only two people at this private concert. As I reminisce about this special performance, I believe there was a kind of magic the pianist brought to the music, a kind of burnish that flowed from mature life experience. Chopin created his waltzes in the early flush of the Romantic Period, and these works reflect the spirit of the times. The waltz she played was incredibly light and quick. As her slender fingers flew over the keys, it was as though the colors and shapes of a well tended flower garden floated through the room. The music lifted me far away from the January morning.

A lovely painting was emerging in my mind, a painting of living roses throwing their gorgeous petals at the sun. There were thorns too on the roses, and there were shadows to give the painting depth. And then it hit me. Part of the artistry of her performance came from her sensitive interpretation and her many years of living.

At the end of the waltz, my pianist smiled at my compliments and quietly mentioned she might have missed a few notes. If she did, I was unaware. And if she did, it only added to the beauty of her interpretation. The performance belonged to both Chopin and to her, and it was, in its way, pure gold!

Shocking Red Lipstick!

Posted on March 1, 2012 by June

My hard working dad was generally very easy going. He loved to perform little tricks to entertain, tricks like magically finding a nickel behind my ear or having a coin suddenly drop out of his nose. He often played his mouth organ for me with great gusto and flourish. I can hardly remember him reprimanding me at all...except for one time. I must have been around 11 or so. It was some time during the middle of WWII and I was spending more and more time staring at myself in the mirror and comparing myself to movie stars. The war had its sexy side: The famous picture of Betty Grable with her curvy back to the camera and looking over her shoulder while smiling flirtatiously at the viewer seemed to be everywhere. The newspaper reported the photo to be in almost every GI's locker, and Betty became known as the No. 1 Pin-up girl of the war. Her beautiful legs were reportedly insured for zillions! Another glamorous Pin-up Girl was Rita Hayworth, a sultry auburn haired beauty whose seductive poses also papered military lockers.

At 11, I was fully grown and often mistaken for being much older. A cute sailor had tried to pick me up when I was riding the merry-go round at Riverview (a large and popular amusement park where my own parents had met). I was getting very conscious of what the newspapers and magazines presented as desirable and I poured over movie magazines, mesmerized by the glamorous stars of stage and screen and often looked into the mirror checking to see what I could do to make myself at least somewhat like them.

For one thing, I learned how to make pin curls, very important for achieving the hairstyles of the day. It took me a while before I mastered twirling my brown hair against my scalp and holding it in place by a bobby pin, but getting the right hair look was crucial in my eyes, and I did not give up. And when some of my classmates began wearing make-up to school, I began trying out my mother's cosmetics and loved how I looked with a popular shade of bright red lipstick.

My very full lips, which I had generally viewed as negative features, suddenly seemed to light up my face...or so I thought. I couldn't wait to show my new look to the world! Everyone would surely be enthralled with the new me! Mom just took it in stride, but when my father came home, he reacted in shock.

My scarlet red lips were not what he wanted to see on his eleven year old daughter. Because I had skipped a grade and a half, I was in 7th grade with older girls, and some were allowed to wear lipstick, but my father would have none of it! It was one of the few times he was really upset by my behavior. Suddenly my fun loving father turned into a forbidding ogre (at least in my eyes). I couldn't understand his reaction for some time. You know how teenagers are. It took a while before I realized that he had my welfare at heart and had thought I was delivering the wrong message.

Eventually dad learned to live with my scarlet lips, as I recall, and I did not become a fallen young woman. We had passed an important milestone.

Coffee, Cream and Me

Posted on May 21, 2012 at 5:58 am

Do these old ears deceive me? Did I hear it right? Coffee, the real thing, straight and not deactivated, is considered good for us?

How can this be? Can this be the same beverage that has been feared by man and woman alike as one that can rev us up to such dangerous levels that it strains our constitutions? Heavens to Betsy! What next?

Can this be the fully octaned coffee that I have learned to approach with care, the same coffee that I stopped offering my guests so that I would not risk the looks of alarm when they found there was no decaf on hand? (Maybe I was overly sensitive, but there were some women who looked very, very concerned.)

Can this be the same coffee that was decaffeinated in both chemical and "natural" ways to such an extent that I read labels religiously before making my purchase? Now that I think about it, I did wonder how removing a natural constituent of a natural bean could be "natural".

End result: I drank mostly regular coffee in private but either one on social occasions.

But now regular coffee has been exonerated. I imagine there are some exceptions, and I am not a doctor, nor am I an expert in the field. However, I was raised to think of coffee as a friend and source of renewed energy. Both mom and dad believed in hard work, and they turned to coffee when they needed to refuel.

They liked it so much and seemed so much cheerier after a cup or two that I asked if I could have some too. I remember they preferred theirs with cream, or rather evaporated milk or "canned milk", as we called it.

My mom was generally easy going when it came to food and beverage, but when it came to coffee, she made it clear that she considered it an adult drink. I did not drink coffee until I was in my teens. When I did, I took it black.

I soon learned black coffee has zero calories, and I came to think of black coffee as the choice of sophisticated adults, and slim and sophisticated was definitely what I wanted to be. When I was in high school I dieted so successfully that I started fainting, and the doctor diagnosed me as having malnutrition. Hard to believe to see me now!

Anyway, for me coffee carries with it a lot of symbolism and memories. Like most people, I've learned not to have so much coffee that it sets me on edge. And as I said before, I am neither an expert nor a doctor, but I'm very glad my cup of Joe in moderation has been given a clean slate!

It's nice to hear on the media that the powers that be think it's actually good for us. I so enjoy it.

I'm "Dancing with the Stars!"

Posted on May 24, 2012 at 5:58 am

I find it a little humorous that people react so strongly when the TV program "Dancing with the Stars" comes up in conversation.

Some openly declare they love to watch it, while others turn up their noses in disdain. I couldn't believe a TV commentator's comment on a morning show upon hearing that Donald Driver rolled around on the floor in jubilation when he was declared this season's winner.

As I recall, she said something like, " It's really only dancing, isn't it?"

Really? As a mother who drove her daughter to ballet lessons for nine years and is herself a devotee of excellence in dance, I strongly disagree. First of all, Driver, although he is a wide receiver on the Green Bay Packers, displays a natural bent for dance, a talent that came to fuller and fuller flower as time went by.

He danced a variety of styles in superb fashion, but he really came into his own in his exuberant country, down home program. The man not only has amazing agility and grace, but his performance sparkled with fun that flew out from the screen.

Upon delving into his background, I learned that family man Driver is also an author of children's books. The books' stories and illustrations are based on his current family life and are meant to amuse and inspire.

This talented man called a U-Haul truck home when he was growing up, and he is reaching out to share his positive views of achieving the American Dream.

In response to an earlier blog, someone cleverly commented that lots of today's problems would be solved if our youth would only stop using "like" as almost every other word in a sentence and also pull their pants up. In his words and in his appearance, Driver lives out the truth that defying convention and speaking in muddled fashion need not be adopted to be successful. We need more role models like him.

Dear Mom, Now I Know

Posted on May 13, 2012
Today is Mother's Day.

I am now 80, and I want to tell you how much I appreciate so many things that you taught me through your words and example.

I thought I had missed out on something when you worked outside the home when it was neither fashionable nor even in most people's lexicon of possibility. I thought I had missed out when things were not as neat and tidy in our apartment as in the homes of my friends.

Life has shown me that you gave me the important things when you made me secure in the knowledge that you thought I was intelligent and attractive and sure to be successful. You were always honest with me, and never talked down to me.

You talked about the challenges of poverty and the value of honest work. Now that times are tough for so many, your pointers on economy become very clearly understandable. So many things you said have taken new meaning over the years. Thank you beautiful mom, thank you for your gift of love.

June

P.S. Happy Mother's Day!

Mother in the Garden

Posted on June 8, 2012 at 12:00 pm

She sat on a chair and held the gushing hose for her rock garden,

The rocks she had gathered over time and carefully aligned

Were holding back the earth...at least mostly.

While I spooned mud in cookie pans, hard at play,

Shaping my slippery cakes of mud and clay,

Me, so proud of them.

She pondered the coal bill now past due...

How much for the milkman? How much for the light?

How much for the meal we'd eat that night?

My mud-cake pans full, I walked to her and asked,

"What is that red flower called?"

"A calla lily, June, my favorite."

The petals looked like fiery tongues to me

Like they'd grown in my fairy tales tempestuously

Scarlet petals a bit darkened, somewhat

wrinkled at their rims,

But its foliage and tall stems provided sturdy limbs

That set it apart.

Mom watered and watered. The air was fragrant with the smell of

wet earth and blossom.

And there was dream in her eye

****

This may be a good place to stop. You see Mom made it clear to me that I was an important part of that dream in her eye. Mom told me about how humiliating it was to be so poor that she took a job cleaning a dentist's floors in order to support herself and her family. She said the dentist made her feel lower than low, and that the pain of his words cut into her soul. Yes, that dentist's words and other humiliations fired up my mother's resolve to live out the American dream with her own blood, sweat and tears.

She wouldn't spend the profits she made owning real estate on herself, however. No matter how I begged her to spend her money on herself, she refused to do so. In her later years, while I was living the life of a typical suburban housewife, she actually bought me clothes that were in her favorite styles and colors. I was uncomfortable with this, but I sure didn't turn them down. She also made it possible for us to purchase our first home.

Now that I am "up in years," I understand a lot of things that used to frustrate me. For much of my life I wanted to fit in and conform to the "June Cleaver", happy and wise, the perfect homemaker image. It wasn't until I went back to school when my children were older that I discovered most of my assumptions about the supposedly perfect family life were largely phantoms of my imagination.

As I pursued my Master's Degree in English Literature, I gained insight into my own true self and came to understand a lot more about those around me, including my remarkable, fiercely determined, and loving mom. Good literature can teach us so much.

My own life style and that of my mother's seem vastly different. Yet as different as our lives might appear, we shared more than a few very basic ideas. Complaining, unless it accomplished something, was a waste of time. Above all she believed life is what we make it. Yes, her really interesting observations and positive attitude live on in my mind to this day. And her unqualified love lives on in my heart.

Be My Love!

When I entered Northwestern University as a sixteen year old, I was as naïve and ill prepared as they come. Actually, I was more than a little rough around the edges. Mom had little interest in socializing, instead totally amercing herself in the management of the six or so apartment buildings that she had acquired through her many years of hard work. More than once she told me how much she loved her life as owner and manager. She never let me forget that she loved me very much too, but I had little exposure to life beyond our home.

Actually, I had little understanding of the prestige attached to a Northwestern degree. So when a boyfriend told me he was going to be married to someone else and I was devastated, I concluded NU was not the place for me. I decided I might have better luck in getting my Mrs. Degree at the University of Illinois in Champaign-Urbana. (Remember, in the 50's most girls went to college for that Mrs. degree!) So, after two years at Northwestern, I transferred to Illinois.

And amazing as it sounds, the very first night I was in Champaign, I went out on a blind date that was arranged by some girls in the house and met my future husband, John. As it turned out, John was from Oak Park, a suburb very close to my home in northwest Chicago. Yet we would never have met had I not gone to Illinois.

The chemistry was electric. So very handsome, I said to myself! Our first date was sealed by smoldering kisses in "the passion pit", an area where we said our goodnights by the front door. This was like the movies. You see, on our first date, my husband to be, of what would become almost 59 years, told me he loved me and wanted to marry me!

I was thrilled by his good looks, so much so that later on I would steal sideway glances at him as he drove, marveling at how much he looked like a movie star. This was what they were always singing about on the radio in those days and now it belonged to me! Mario Lanza's hit song, "Be My Love", was played everywhere throughout the country and became our own "special song." I love that I can listen to Mario Lanza's recording even today and share the beautiful lyrics with the grandchildren.

We were crazy in love and thought the song had been written for us. Unlike today, we lived when the idea of the perfect romance was considered cool and a very real possibility. We were lucky, we had found our love.

John graduated before me and we wrote each other love letters, letters that show how much we missed one another. I treasure them.

And this is how we met and began a life together, a life of almost 59 years of rainbows and passionate kisses and storm clouds, a life that included the heartaches and sweet times of our long life together. Life had a lot to teach us and we grew up together during our marriage... if any of us really totally grows up. We both changed over the years. But underneath it all was a sense of mutual respect and until the very end, an undying passion. Together we raised four children and lived to see 13 grandchildren, living out the promise of our evolving but everlasting love.

www.ingramcontent.com/pod-product-compliance
Lightning Source LLC
Chambersburg PA
CBHW051431280526
45785CB00003B/1240